HOW TO BE WELL

Praise for *How To Be Well*

'At once an exposé of beauty and wellness trends, a critique of patriarchal culture, and a guide for individuals seeking real wellness not by purchasing things but by developing inner resources and making sustainable choices, this is the detox many people need from, well, detoxes and their often-detrimental effects' **Library Journal**

'Penetrating and thought-provoking, this will cause readers to think twice before reaching for the latest purported cure-all' **Publishers Weekly**

'Readers will find lots of informative and entertaining food (or juice) for thought' **Booklist**

'A magical synthesis of crackerjack reporting, incisive cultural commentary, and, most importantly, elegant, self-reflective memoir, *How to Be Well* perfectly captures the defining ethos of our day' **Joanna Rakoff, author of** *My Salinger Year*

'Amy Larocca brings her buoyant wit, cultural fluency, and indispensable skepticism to this rollicking exploration of our desperation for wellness, our devotion to CBD, self-care, and Soul Cycle, deftly separating the gobbledygook from the truly transformative' **Ariel Levy, author of** *The Rules Do Not Apply*

'Larocca's tour is a lively one, full of information and humor' **New York Times**

'Authoritative and witty, personal without being chummy' **New York Times**

Amy Larocca

HOW TO BE WELL

Finding a way through the
self-care epidemic without losing
your mind and your money

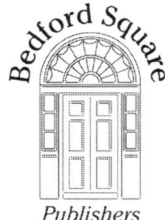

First published in the US in 2025 by Alfred A. Knopf, a division of
Penguin Random House LLC,
New York, USA

First published in the UK in 2026 by Bedford Square Publishers Ltd,
London, UK

@bedfordsq.publishers

A Maxim Jakubowski book
© Amy Larocca, 2025

The right of Amy Larocca to be identified as the author of this work has been asserted in accordance with the Copyright, Designs and Patents Act 1988. All rights reserved. No part of this book may be reproduced, stored in or introduced into a retrieval system, or transmitted, in any form or by any means (electronic, mechanical, photocopying, recording or otherwise) without the written permission of the publishers.

Any person who does any unauthorised act in relation to this publication may be liable to criminal prosecution and civil claims for damages.
A CIP catalogue record for this book is available from the British Library.

ISBN
978-1-83501-432-5 (Trade paperback)
978-1-83501-433-2 (eBook)

2 4 6 8 10 9 7 5 3 1

Typeset in 12.75 on 16.25pt Bembo Std
by Avocet Typeset, Bideford, Devon, EX39 2BP
Printed and bound in Great Britain by
CPI Group (UK) Ltd, Croydon CR0 4YY

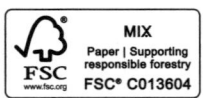

The manufacturer's authorised representative in the EU for product safety is Easy Access System Europe, Mustamäe tee 50, 10621 Tallinn, Estonia
gpsr.requests@easproject.com

For Will, Oona, and Ruby

CONTENTS

Introduction	9
PART I: CURE	25
Medicine and Its Alternatives	33
Holistic, Functional, Profitable	40
Kooks	57
Chronic Illness	72
Self-Care	78
PART II: GLOW	87
Body Positive?	95
Sex Positive	103
Clean Beauty	107
Dressing to Be Well	111
Glow Lifestyle	120
PART III: SPIRIT AND SOUL	127
Soul	132
Exercise	141
Self-Love	150
Cult	157
Outside of Exercise	162

Contents

PART IV: PURE	167
Cleanse	174
Environment	188
All Natural	196
Politics	200
Vaccines and the Rabbit Hole	206
Cleaning as Rite	214
PART V: BEYOND	219
Meditation/Mindfulness	223
Tripping	237
What About Men?	242
Biohacking	248
Immortality	262
Conclusion	271
Acknowledgments	279
Notes	283
Index	303
About the Author	319

INTRODUCTION

Do you know a well woman? Odds are you do. She is everywhere with her clean, clear skin, sipping from a nontoxic container full of an expensive, mysterious broth. She is the friend who is not religious but is spiritual; she swears by her Transcendental Meditation practice. She swears by a lot of things, like a very specific whisk for her matcha that she sourced from a very specific ethical, artisanal website. She is educated, but not rigid in thought. She is a seeker, and she is unashamed of her frailties because she is so actively engaged in finding unique solutions and cures. You might know her only virtually, but she shares enough about herself for you to understand that she is simultaneously ambitious and content, that her boundaries and orgasms and poop are all firm and beautifully formed. She has so much advice on how you might be more like her, with her working definition of 'tincture' and her pretty pill case full of pretty pills. She is beautiful, tranquil, fertile, productive. She is pure of intention, heavy metals, food dyes, and dread.

The well woman was ready with her vitamin D supplements, her soothing breathwork, and her slip-on shearling Birkenstock clogs during the last pandemic, and she'll be ready for the next one, too. Every generation of American women has had to wrestle with an imaginary ideal, some caricature of femininity to chase and, crucially, to buy. The wasp-waisted housewife

Introduction

practiced at thrift and the roasting of big joints of meat; the so-called power women, in mannish shoulder pads and floppy silk ties, succeeding in the boardroom and the bedroom – bringing home the bacon, frying it up in a pan, and so on.

What all these ideal American women have in common is that they are always very thin and they do not complain, no matter how many responsibilities are added to their list.

Today's ideal woman is the well woman, hopped up on her plant-based diet and elaborate adaptogen regimen, clear-eyed from her spectacular sleep hygiene and Transcendental Meditation and, maybe, just a touch of psychedelics. She might appear, at first glance, to be an improvement on her idealized predecessors – all that 'self-care' – but look a little closer, and she is alarmingly the same. She's a whiz in the kitchen, a master of time management, a source of spirituality, selflessness, industriousness, and calm. She folds her T-shirts into thirds; she starts and ends each day in gratitude.

And her pores, her lovely pores, are undetectable to the naked eye.

It was in pursuit of becoming a well woman that I found myself white-knuckled and curled up like a baby shrimp, naked from the waist down, on a crooked exam table in a basement office on Manhattan's far West Side one chilly December afternoon.

The colonic is the flossing of the wellness world: a means of getting rid of the filth your regular routine might miss, all the filth you cannot see. Flossing, however, is not controversial.

My doctor had told me not to do this ('*whyyyy?*' was how she put it), as had the more credible corners of the internet. The risks ranged from rectal perforation to dehydration to worse, but some number of people, and some other corners of the internet, had promised it would change my life, provide perspective and purpose and a near-ecstatic lightness of being. One woman told me that colonics make her feel as if she can *fly*, that rinsing out the nooks and crannies of her colon was like rinsing out the corners of her psyche. What emerged was not just normal fecal waste you'd expect, but also a lifetime of insecurities and sadness, major and minor. I lay there, cramped and longing to rejoin the vertical axis, while for thirty minutes a friendly enough ex-nurse named Diane vigorously flushed my guts with (I hope) sterile water, everything exiting via flexible rubber tube.

I stayed very, very still, counted backward from a hundred, and tried to focus on my breath and everything I would like to be rid of:

potential pandemics
climate change
several justices of the Supreme Court (and the people they married)
   five to seven perimenopausal pounds, largely concentrated
     around the bra line
the slow and inevitable downhill march to death

I didn't want to just walk out of Diane's office into my own, familiar reality; I wanted to fly, specifically into a different, kinder, gentler place.

It's a lot to ask of the contents of my bowels, but it feels as though Diane's table and tubes, and their many parallel setups, are being asked something like it by an ever-growing number of people every day as wellness expands across the culture like a rash.

Wellness is currently a $5.6 trillion industry according to the Global Wellness Institute, and it is growing faster than the rest of the economy. McKinsey & Company reports that investment in digital health start-ups reached record highs in 2021: $29 billion across 730 deals, compared with $15 billion across 480 deals just a year before. That's a tremendous number of wearable monitors and organic eye cream and mushroom

INTRODUCTION

teas to navigate, but these are the ideas informing not only how we spend but also how we eat, sleep, think, worry, and dream. Wellness is the modern ideal of womanhood that we are measured, and measure ourselves, against. And it doesn't appear to be letting up.

Feeling better is the overwhelming desire not only of my generation as we hit midlife, and whatever gray state comes next, but also of my daughters' generation, who are young enough to sleep like still-buried potatoes and to then wake up bright-eyed no matter the antics of the day before.

It is of course easy to scoff at Diane and her nasty tubes, and at the golden vitamin tablets I order from England and take every day at tremendous cost with dubious result, and at the idea of paying to submerge myself in a giant bucket of ice, which I have also, on occasion, done. But the pressure to take these extra measures feels great. I increasingly find myself willing to choke down the healthy sardines, relax into child's pose, review the teachings of Joseph Pilates with an open and earnest mind.

I know a lot about aspiration; I have a strong understanding of want. For twenty years I worked full-time as a fashion journalist: my topic was what people wear and why they wear it, parsing the lines of internal and external forces that lead us to choose *that* shoe, *those* pants, *that* dress. I have spent a great deal of my life puzzling over the difficult messages our culture sends women about who we are supposed to want to be. I traveled a lot, often to European capitals to watch a long stream of fashion shows, as well as the hyperactive peacocking outside the venue doors, or to spend hours interviewing designers in their workrooms, wandering cities with them as they revealed their inspirations and muse. I know the craft: I understand proportion, construction, and silhouette, but my real expertise is in the *longing* at fashion's core. Fashion is about beauty, of course, but it is also about the desire to elevate daily life from its more banal limitations, to consciously and actively share something about how you'd like to be perceived by the rest of the world.

And it can also be about wanting things that are difficult to get. Fashion shows used to be assiduously private. Designer clothing was prohibitively expensive and hard to access outside a few key cities. To know about and access fashion was something elite. To belong to something mostly hidden from view was a tremendous part of its appeal.

But over the course of my time in that industry, fashion grew ever more democratic. Shows were streamed online; what we saw in those rooms was simultaneously available all over the world. People could watch from their basements; they could watch in their tatty sweatpants and robes! The relationships this access built between old brands and new customers meant that it was in the brands' best interest to make more and more merchandise available via diverse platforms. If you live on a farm in Indiana and you want a Gucci dress, you can get that dress hand-delivered to your doorstep, probably the very next day. And if you can't afford a Gucci dress, Gucci probably has a key fob or a lipstick or a T-shirt in closer reach.

Waiting for shows to start and sharing rides between them, my fashion friends and I often talked about which shows we'd liked, what from the runway we could imagine owning for ourselves. But we also talked increasingly about our health, our wellness: our vitamins, supplements, energy healers, and gyms. We talked about where to buy green juice in Milan. There were certain yoga teachers in Paris who would come do private sessions at the Ritz; there was an ex-ballerina who did lengthening sessions in a pretty apartment she'd rent for the week, and a square-jawed trainer who organized early morning runs in the Tuileries.

It was a whole new culture of elitism. Only a certain tier of photographers and designers and editors knew to spend their

Introduction

free time and money at Vivamayr, a famous Austrian fasting spa that one friend calls 'the Bum Spa,' with a haunted look in her eye. Only certain stylists have the cell number for Dr Passler, a Greenwich Village nutritionist/chiropractor who's big into biofeedback. If you know, though, you can tell who does when you spot them eating a certain Hudson Valley goat cheese by the log.

In a now-legendary interview with *Elle* magazine in 2015, the glamorous California juice bar owner Amanda Chantal Bacon recounted what she eats in a single day. The following is her early morning routine:

> I usually wake up at 6:30am, and start with some Kundalini meditation and a 23-minute breath set – along with a copper cup of silver needle and calendula tea – before my son Rohan wakes... At 8am, I have a warm, morning chi drink on my way to the school drop off, drunk in the car! It contains more than 25 grams of plant protein, thanks to vanilla mushroom protein and stone ground almond butter, and also has the super endocrine, brain, immunity, and libido-boosting powers of Brain Dust, cordyceps, reishi, maca, and Shilajit resin. I throw ho shou wu and pearl in as part of my beauty regime. I chase it with three quinton shots for mineralization and two lipospheric vitamin B-complex packets for energy.

It was a whole new vocabulary for aspiration, a whole new category for want: *Cordyceps* and *ho shou wu* replacing Valentino and Prada as esoteric and chic and desirably hard to get.

Many of my friends and acquaintances from the fashion world fully switched streams. A stylist I'd worked with on a cover shoot became a wellness coach and drank her own still-warm placenta in a smoothie live on Instagram hours after giving birth. The owner of a shop where I used to buy short dresses and thick tights when I was into that sort of thing was diagnosed with celiac disease and then turned her business into a 'clean beauty' destination with rose quartz embedded under the floorboards. 'The vibrations,' she promised, 'are great.' (She also coauthored a book with recommendations for achieving 'high vibrational beauty,' with a recipe for a 'Spring Has Sprung Kombucha Frappe,' and another for roast potatoes inspired by the aesthetics of the minimalist architect John Pawson.) The party girl known for her leather miniskirts got long-term, chronic Lyme disease: her *New York Times* marriage announcement described the radical bee venom therapies that she credits with bringing her back to health, as well as her dairy-and-gluten-free wedding banquet held at a Sonoma vineyard. The retailer of expensive clothes to wear to expensive bars sold it all and opened a meditation studio with gentle, Turrell-inspired lighting in a dome. My friend the accessories editor pursued an online degree in nutrition, and when a glamorous makeup artist came for dinner, she sent a loaf of gluten-free bread and a tub of unpasteurized butter in thanks.

On Instagram, I follow Rosemary Ferguson, who was one of the most iconic models of London's glamorous 1990s, the era of so-called heroin chic. Ferguson was discovered in a McDonald's on Oxford Street and went on to be in British *Vogue* and *The Face* and to star in the original Miu Miu advertising campaign. Her best friend is Kate Moss, and she's married to the artist Jake Chapman – none of which suggests a life of spirulina. But now she lives in rural Gloucestershire and works as a nutritionist; she leads virtual 'reset programs' that are all about cold showers and hot soup. I also follow Alexandra Golovanoff, a Parisian ex-model and cashmere sweater designer who details the yoga retreats she takes with the designer Julie de Libran, the Paris *Vogue* editor Mélanie Huynh, and Isabella Capece Galeota, an executive at the Louis Vuitton Foundation and the founder

Introduction

of Maisie Café, a fashionable, organic, vegan, and gluten-free place just off the Place de la Concorde.

Golovanoff makes them the best-ever yoga outfits for their trips.

And they are all capable of perfect inversion.

The elephant in the room is Gwyneth Paltrow, ur-wellness she-god embodying mega-success and abundant, extravagant, romantic self-love. In the fifteen years since Paltrow started Goop as a weekly newsletter offering travel tips for her rich friends, she's gone so far into wellness that she's claimed credit for the popularity of yoga, introduced the concept of the wellness divorce, and turned sex toys into mainstream instruments of health.

Goop's $250 million piece of the market, rife as it is with hypocrisies, manipulations, and sometimes even big fat lies, makes a lot of noise and gets a lot of attention, but it's only the tip of the iceberg. Wellness is on shelves all over the country, in venues both rarefied and mass. Walmart has an annual Wellness Day and Costco publishes a quarterly health magazine called *Healthy Living*. Dunkin' Donuts has introduced its own take on avocado toast.

I sometimes think of wellness as the project of buying your own body back for yourself, a world in which the branded, luxury version of YOU is available for sale, a bizarre arrangement that comes with the side effect of exposing some of the greatest inequities in modern American life. The offer seems to be this: with the right combination of determination, access, interest, and money, an elevated state is attainable, reasonable, logical. It's what we all should aspire to and for.

The climb toward these goals is frequently accompanied by the gentle buzz of a lite-FM spirituality, an idea about being that offers something like a religion — in this case, the gospel of infinite possibilities of the self — to a population of secular seekers also interested in multitasking, burning calories as much as finding connection, and soothing their lonely and frightened souls.

Many of the ideas we call wellness aren't new, but their ascendance in both the culture and the economy has been as enormous as it has been quick. These are theories, methods, practices, and hypotheses that have been around for eons, and often it's just the packaging and the marketing and the interpretations that are new. Consider, for example, the case of kale. Before 2012, the biggest consumer of the chewy, cabbagey leaf was Pizza Hut, which did not serve it but instead used it as a decorative garnish on its salad bars. In 2013, a New York-based English publicist named Oberon Sinclair told reporters that she'd been hired by the 'American Kale Association' to 'make kale cool,' and a slew of articles soon followed. At its peak, Beyoncé herself appeared in a 'Kale' sweatshirt. Sinclair finally admitted that she made the whole thing up. She just wanted to see how far she could push an idea. 'I'm a punk at heart,' she said, when busted. But also: 'I've always loved kale! It's an amazing vegetable!'

The case of kale was a harmless prank – it is a highly nutritious vegetable, rich in vitamins K, C, A, and B, not to mention carotenoids, lutein, folate, and fiber! – but often the repurposing and reselling of old ideas is followed by accusations of cultural and historical appropriation. This quest to be better and feel better is as old as time, the ultimate human riddle, but there's no question that this current wave has become a tsunami, one that swells in inverse proportion to what too often feels like the end of the world. Maybe it began with the smartphone – all that endless information, all those photos of things too horrible to imagine, beeping and reminding us all day long, confronting us in our most private and intimate spaces and times. Could we have predicted the wellness movement when it became possible to watch GoPro videos off a soldier's helmet the day after a bloody attack? There is no question the

Introduction

movement is connected to politics. When Donald Trump was elected in 2016, Instagram posts labeled #selfcare, and its close relatives #selfcareisntselfish, #selfcareishealthcare, #selfcareobsessed, and #radicalselfcare, increased exponentially: within a year the number had gone up ninefold, which means that by 2020 there were more than twenty million photographs on the app of bath-tubs and acai, bowls of porridge, honey yogurt face masks, and inspirational quotations like 'self-care is how you take your power back.' The pandemic exploded this trend yet again four years later when consistent public guidance was hard to find, and harder to trust. COVID ended up delivering the hard proof and validation that wellness's greatest pitches have long sought. In so-called peacetimes, these habits and rituals might seem silly or overblown, but how quickly 'self-care' went from seeming self-indulgent to just plain smart.

Even in the face of unavoidable facts about what makes a person well (it's privilege), for the body workers and colon therapists, the functional medicine women and men, the Transcendental Meditators and the supplement gobblers, the spiritual gangsters and the Moon Juicers... this was it. The rapture. They were, kind of, right about everything. Taking care of yourself was going to be the only way to get through our terrifying new world.

In my mission to make some sense of how we got here and what it means to have this abstracted wellness she-god as the feminine ideal, I met with all sorts of people across the spectrum of earnest, wacky, and woo-woo. That colonic was not my only excursion into the dubious and unpleasant. I've ingested gallons of thick, unsweetened green (and brown) juices and broths; I've purged and cleansed my closet, my consciousness, my gut. I've wrapped myself up like a burrito and sweated until I felt that my heart might pop, frozen myself blue in a person-sized walk-in fridge. I've mailed vials of my blood and saliva and pee to mysterious laboratories in far-off states, all in search of problems I hadn't even considered I might have. I have spent so much money on tinctures, teas, gels, and pills – I've spent ridiculous money on collagen juice on the very same day that I read dozens of articles explaining exactly why it doesn't work. I might buy some more later today.

I've met a lot of extremely savvy entrepreneurs grabbing at the tentacles of this ever-booming industry that just grows and expands with no limits. I have watched large American enterprises attempt to shift to seemingly impossible positions: Philip Morris, the company that brought America the Marlboro Man, launched a campaign, this time to 'unsmoke' the world.

I've also met a lot of people genuinely frightened about the state of American well-being and health. When wellness is silly and costs a lot – cow cuddling, goat yoga, GP's vagina steaming, her vagina rocks, her vagina candles, not to mention her rectal ozone insufflation – it is easy to dismiss. With every stick of palo santo incense sold, the problem that good health in America has been elevated as a luxury commodity as opposed to a fundamental right is further obscured. Women are the targets of so much misleading information, so much shaming, and so many superstitions that we like to think we've abandoned but are now touted as progressive, helpful, even feminist. What makes the whole thing ever trickier is that sometimes – and only sometimes – they are these things, too.

It's a brew that has the potential to drive you nuts.

The well woman is no longer a secret to the privileged few: she is an aspiration of the mainstream. Like the cerulean sweater from *The Devil Wears Prada* that made its slow descent from the Paris runway to an Old Navy near you, being 'well' is now big, mainstream, and for sale at the strip mall next door.

At my local drugstore, which is part of a national chain, a giant green disk reading 'WELLNESS' hangs above the aisles in an attempt to ascribe higher purpose to the same old

Introduction

Gursky-esque selection of plastic-bottled mouthwash, animal-tested lip gloss, and Band-Aids and aspirin and steroid sprays for a stuffy nose. Street-level storefronts are filling disproportionately with boutique-style doctors' offices, all shiny marble countertops, free kombucha, and Berber rugs. These doctor brands have beautifully designed logos and charismatic leaders who write manuals and books and host podcasts featuring celebrity guests. They produce their own, for-profit lines of supplements and shakes and foam rollers, and sometimes you'll get the unsettling message: your doctor is having a *sale*. Health at a discount, wellness at a rate.

We all know vulnerability, are all confronted at different points in our lives with the fragility of our whole enterprise. I have lost too many friends, at this point, to causes that have been called avoidable and also unavoidable. It's a distinction that has very little, if any, meaning in the end.

My husband and I have two daughters, and our younger daughter was born extremely *un*well, with a large tumor crowding her airway and obliterating her ability to breathe. The tumor had grown fast and late – it was not apparent on the many anatomy scans and sonograms I'd had – we found out in the delivery room, and then she was whisked away in a heated Perspex pod placed in the back of an ambulance that sped up the highway to a big hospital uptown. It was against hospital policy to move me – freshly stitched up from a C-section – with her, so she went with my husband while kind nurses pumped sedatives into the IV that was already in my arm and I lay there: frantic, tearful, and foggy. Once we were all reunited, the doctors told us that what had happened was a lightning strike, an anomaly. Her tumor – a cluster of undifferentiated cells known as a teratoma, or a 'vanishing twin' – was not genetic, and it was benign. 'Good' luck following quickly on the tail of bad. She was cured with a long, complicated surgery and several months of inpatient recovery involving intubation and tube feedings, followed by months of therapies at home.

'It's not your fault,' the doctors told us, and we nodded politely in response to the scientific explanations, but then late at night, and even still, I find myself wondering what, exactly, I had done. Did I use the wrong liner on my shower curtain, sleep on the wrong mattress, pad barefoot across the wrong rug? Was this because I gave in to a first trimester craving for the ten-piece McNuggets, inhaled in one single, selfish bite, hormones and additives and preservatives and all? During the months I spent by her Isolette, I listened to NICU nurses describe the differences in breast milk quality offered by different mothers. The mothers who ate fast and processed foods and soda were said to have thin yellow milk, which they said was even less nutritionally useful than the smelly, sticky, powdery formula we were taught to disdain. It quickly became clear that this was a class distinction. But when the issue at hand is the survival of your kid, you become desperate to be on the right side of the line, whatever your politics. If the expensive magical breathing of Pilates and monounsaturated avocado fat and the ritual chanting of a Vedic mantra would help me produce the thick, creamy elixir that might carry our baby to nice rosy health, I was in.

In motherhood I was so gullible, so vulnerable. I was just so *desperate*. It is likely that all of it – from the McNuggets I did eat to all the processed white bread I didn't – is just a form of indulgent superstition, salt thrown over the shoulder, the greatest placebo of all time. What matters is what also got me through COVID: the cumulative effect of a diet rich in whole, nutritious foods, a lifetime of nights spent in safe, clean places, access to good doctors, fresh air, and water consistently untainted by poison and lead. But both then and now, even with everything I know, I do not claim to rise above the wellness industry's many seductive promises, above the pressure I feel to

Introduction

embody this latest ideal. This is a book about women, because wellness is mostly an industry by and for women, just as the diet and beauty industries it seeks to replace are.

It feels irresponsible to be satisfied with 'fine,' and even when I am, I wonder if some higher level of health is available, and if the pursuit of such a thing is narcissism or entertainment, harmless or something worse? I weigh myself every morning and reflect on how many of the dieting habits that I was once taught were necessary to successful, mainstream white American womanhood are now sold to me as 'self-care.'

I don't have diabetes – I don't even have prediabetes – but I leaped at the chance to wear a continuous glucose monitor (CGM), basically for kicks.

This book isn't a guide, but you are welcome to use it that way: by the time you're done reading, you'll know what ashwagandha is, have a working understanding of how mindfulness works, and understand why the fanciest vacation you can take involves going to Ibiza for a hit of psychedelic toad administered by a once-famous celebrity shoe designer who is something of a shaman now.

This is an attempt to understand how and why we are here, how wellness moves across the landscape of the concrete – the medical care we seek and receive, the way we spend our money and hope to appear to the people we meet – into aspects far less easy to touch. Is wellness just consumerism, or is it a new politics, a new religion? Today on my way to work I listened to a podcast about the first subdivision in outer space, which should be built before my daughters are thirty years old, so maybe we do live in a world where one might have the option, as an increasing number of people predict and now sell, to indefinitely delay or postpone death.

Nothing really changed for me on that December afternoon in Diane's basement lair. I spent the evening with a terrible case of the cramps and feeling a bit absurd. For the next few weeks, though, I did experience the slightest sensation of lightness as I moved through my life. It wasn't much, or it was imagined, but so what. There it was! If nothing terrible happens in the course of a wellness experiment, because you are always dealing with a sample size of one, it's hard to know what you'd feel like without the chunks of frozen cauliflower and three varieties of seeds (chia, hemp, flax) in a disgusting breakfast shake, or to remember how cheap, trippy cough syrup feels in place of spoonfuls of honey from $80 jars that come direct from New Zealand. So why not call it good?

Even after all this research, even with everything I know, I can still shock myself by how vulnerable I am, how easily I measure myself against this imagined well ideal. It's far too easy to abandon logic, reason, and common sense in search of the soothing sensation that I have any control over anything at all, that if only I pay enough attention, I might become her, that if I try hard enough I might wear the protective cloak of someone who is, finally, *truly well*.

PART I
CURE

IN ORDER TO HAVE WELLNESS, we must first name its opposite, and its opposite is not necessarily disease. It's the state of being *un*well, and it takes many different forms.

A 2022 marketing campaign for Sollis Health (pronounced 'solace'), a boutique urgent care medical practice with offices in New York City, the Hamptons, California, and Palm Beach, shared the struggles of client 'warriors' including the actresses Freida Pinto, who suffered postpartum depression, and Alyssa Milano, who has anxiety, and the Victoria's Secret model Martha Hunt, who has been managing scoliosis since she was fourteen. It turns out the successful comedian Nick Kroll has bad allergies and sometimes performs with hives on his neck, and the *Baywatch* movie actress Charlotte McKinney has interstitial cystitis. Sloane Crosley, successful writer and girl-about-town, has Ménière's disease, which is a disorder of the inner ear.

These are all manifestations of unwellness – which is to say, all under the umbrella of ailments that are disruptive without being life-threatening and that wellness culture proclaims to be able to treat.

Sollis Health's long roster of beautiful people is also classic wellness culture. The average ER in America has a ninety-minute waiting time; at Sollis it's unusual to wait longer than five minutes. You can also opt for a house call and spend any waiting time leafing through your own Yayoi Kusama monograph in your own Desmond & Dempsey pajamas, drinking your own antioxidant blends. The luxury of voicing and treating discomfort is just a question of cost.

All of which is to say, when it comes to health, the entire wellness industry rides on a set of uncomfortable contradictions. Better to name than ignore, but also who is allowed to name their suffering, and who is believed when they do? When are we thinking creatively about chronic illness, and when are we crowdsourcing snake oil sales pitches? When are we expanding our narrow, often discriminatory definition of medicine, and when are we somaticizing the ordinary unhappiness of being alive?

When I was a child, a case of homesickness on a sleepover was managed with a fictional stomachache and a late-night SOS call home. The kids we host are comfortable describing not only their food allergies but also their food sensitivities and the special products they require for sleep: melatonin gummies, soothing orb-like lights, plug-in devices that mimic sounds of rivers, cicadas, whales. Whatever else unwellness is, it's a spectrum.

The problems described are both physical and emotional, and they tend not to be life-threatening in the short term. They are the problems that people have historically ignored, managed, succumbed to, and suffered from mostly in private.

There's a popular, sentimental fantasy, or myth, about the old-school American 'family doctor' – invariably a man with a leather bag who cared for multiple generations, delivering babies in the beginning and gently shutting the lids at the end. These avuncular, familiar, often mustachioed MDs were not concerned with HMOs and did not flirt with pharmaceutical sales reps in their flashy cars or dabble in supplement pyramid schemes. Their treatment of patients was based as much on experience and intuition as on any sort of generally accepted medical practice. They were no-nonsense, they were all-knowing, they had all the answers.

Like so many ideas about earlier Americas, this is a fiction. Even when some version of this scenario did exist, it was for the benefit of the very few; health care in America has historically neglected large segments of the population – women, always, but also racial and ethnic minorities and anyone unable to pay. Lamenting 'the way it used to be' fails to consider the colossal number of people who never got what they needed.

The standard and method of care that most Americans now consider 'normal' medicine begin in the early part of the twentieth century, the result of a 1910 report commissioned by the Carnegie Foundation. The purpose of the report was to evaluate the state of American medical education; to conduct it, the foundation hired an educator named Abraham Flexner, who was not a doctor or a scientist, but had recently completed a study of the country's public education system. Flexner visited all 150 of the medical schools then operating in America and singled out Johns Hopkins in Baltimore, which was, he said, the model for what medical education should look like: clean, clinical, data-based – *allopathic*. Flexner encouraged the universal adoption of scientific knowledge and its advancement as the ethos of the profession: concrete answers with data to back it all up. Anything softer – osteopathy, say, or nutrition, which was considered relevant when Flexner began – was disparaged when the professions failed to produce quantifiable results.

Flexner's report proposed a lot of changes, many of which are undeniably good – he called for drastic improvements in hygiene, for example – but its insistence on a solution-based ideal with the goal of solving acute problems meant that the onus of 'cause' was not considered the doctor's problem to solve, or even consider. Flexner did not believe that lifestyle changes had a place in medicine. That was something for somewhere else, something for the rich, the weak, the lonely.

Some of the roots of a lot of the inequities in modern health care are also presaged in the Flexner report. Flexner believed, for example, that Black doctors should primarily serve Black communities and educate them on hygienic practices, lest they infect whites with contagious disease. When he did see a role for Black Americans in the larger medical world, it was in a position of subservience to their white counterparts. Medical education was segregated in the South, and only two Black medical schools (Howard University College of Medicine and Meharry Medical College) survived the publication of the report, and for the next fifty years these two institutions educated three-quarters of the nation's Black doctors.

There were relatively few women studying medicine at the time Flexner wrote his report, and this absence manifested itself in medical trials for decades. A lot of the research and testing that has informed American standard medical practice has been done exclusively on men: for example, the first twenty years of the Baltimore Longitudinal Study of Aging, which began in 1958, and the 1982–89 study that suggested that a daily aspirin might prevent heart disease, and the 1973–82 Multiple Risk Factor Intervention Trial – MRFIT – that looked at the effects of dietary change and smoking cessation on heart disease. Even most lab rats are male. A study done in the early 1960s that looked at whether hormone supplementation after menopause could affect heart health was, puzzlingly, conducted entirely on men. (The outcome was that millions of women in the 1970s were prescribed postmenopausal estrogen supplements.) In 1986, a study on the relationship between obesity and estrogen activity, and the risk of developing breast and uterine cancer, had only male subjects. Olympia Snowe, a congresswoman at the time, said, 'Somehow, I find it hard to believe that the male-dominated medical community would tolerate a study of prostate cancer that used only women as research subjects.'

In 1910, only 6 percent of doctors in the United States were female. By 1960, that percentage had not budged. The New York Obstetrical Society did not have any women members and held its meetings at the Yale Club in Manhattan, which at the time did not even allow women inside. It was not until the 1970s with a class-action complaint by the Women's Equity Action League against every university – including every medical school in the United States – and the 1972 passage of Title IX (which prohibited discrimination on the basis of sex in any educational institution receiving federal funds) that things started to change: by 1976 the proportion of women in medical school was 24 percent, or four times what it had been in 1960. Women now make up more than 50 percent of American medical students. The enrollment of Black students in medical school has also been rising – in 2022, 10 percent of matriculants were Black – but presently only 5.7 percent of practicing American medical doctors are Black.

The result of Flexner's legacy, as well as the many disciples of clinical, *DSM*-driven allopathy, is a medical establishment with a narrow view of what constitutes both illness and treatment, and an inequitable understanding of patients who aren't white and/or male. 'One of the bitterest aspects of my illnesses has been this: not only did I suffer from a disease, but I suffered at the hands of a medical establishment that, for too long, failed to fully credit my testimony,' Meghan O'Rourke has written of seeking treatment for a complex set of chronic conditions. 'The U.S. medical system not only failed to diagnose me; it stopped my quest in its tracks.'

The tests we take and the diagnoses we receive have become the standard, accepted measure of whether or not we are sick. 'I got the test results,' you might announce, 'and therein lies the truth about my health.' Or 'I will take these medications, and then I will no longer be unwell.' What this discounts is how patients actually feel, how they experience the reality of their suffering. As Sarah Ramey points out in her memoir, *The Lady's Handbook for Her Mysterious Illness,* if a test fails to figure out the problem, it is not the test that is the problem; it is the patient.

And of course, in the old model we go looking only when something goes wrong; our most common relationship to health is reactive. Proactive measures, like dieting and 'health food,' are considered mostly cosmetic.

When some people say wellness, this is what they mean: a movement that protests the lockstep rigidity of traditional Western medicine, that attempts to make people feel better on a cell-deep level, that seeks to harness the accumulated knowledge of thousands of years of medical exploration for *everyone* and figure out how not to feel so crap. But that's a tall order. The results have brought us, among other things, an evolving cultural definition of 'health,' holistic medicine entering the mainstream, a swell of immensely profitable boutique treatment options, an internet universe of forums and testimonies, an influential slate of celebrity doctors and gurus, and a whole lot of weird stuff to either put in or cleanse from your body.

As it goes with such enormous goals, the results are mixed.

MEDICINE AND ITS ALTERNATIVES

In 1979, when *60 Minutes* was the top-rated television program in America, the middle-aged correspondent Dan Rather took on an emergent topic. 'Wellness,' he said, arching his brow skeptically north. 'There's a word you don't hear every day.'

Rather's bemused report was about people taking an active approach to their health, noting that one doctor calls it 'recognizing that health is not simply the absence of disease.' It is, instead, something else: the practice of individuals diagnosing and treating themselves when traditional doctors can't or won't address their aches, their pains, their assorted sufferings and maladies.

Rather's segment focused on a self-care program at the Wellness Resource Center in Northern California (natch), founded by the seriously bearded Dr John Travis.

Health, Dr Travis said, 'was not the absence of sickness' but 'an ongoing, dynamic state of growth.'

'Just because you aren't sick,' he said, 'you don't have any symptoms, you could go get a checkup and then get a clean bill of health, doesn't mean you are well.'

Rather asks a group of health professionals who are learning about wellness from Dr Travis if they are serving 'a middle-class cult.'

Please, they say, raising their eyebrows right back.

Medicine and Its Alternatives

'In wellness,' one of them explains, 'you are the leader. You're your own guru. And you're the perfect person who is just trying to make your life better and more full.'

What Rather's report implied was that spending too much time or money on this was an indulgence, something silly, something for people with more money and time than sense. He was a mouthpiece for the skepticism of his mainstream upper-middle-class audience, who lumped these ideas in with a general distaste for anything countercultural. Flexnerian medicine focused so strongly on testable and quantifiable data. This wellness stuff was... soft. It was woo-woo. It was something that should probably stay in California. As Woody Allen says in *Annie Hall*, which had come out two years earlier, 'There's wheat germ killers out here!' (Later, at a Hollywood restaurant, Allen consults his menu and sadly orders 'alfalfa sprouts and a plate of mashed yeast.') When I was young and newly employed, my job offered health insurance, and I was able to opt in. I went to doctors who took my company's plan, but my company changed plans frequently in search of better deals, so I changed doctors all the time, recounting my medical history over and over to people I was unlikely to see again. I didn't hugely mind: I was young and healthy and had come of age in the callous and capitalist 1980s in a wealthy New York suburb where many parents (not mine) worked on Gordon Gekko-era Wall Street and voted for both Ronald Reagan and George H. W. Bush. The doctor was for annual physicals and the as-needed swab for strep throat, the free-and-easy prescribing of liquid antibiotics and tiny tubes of eye-drops for pinkeye.

'Health' was something to do with Tab soda, Jane Fonda, and the occasional dose of mild(ish) amphetamines, which came over the counter branded as diet pills, illustrated by narrow waists and measuring tapes. The emphasis was on how you looked rather than how you felt. I can still hear Jane Fonda's voice explaining 'how we get rid of the wobbly wobble!' of arm fat; my friends and I did videos after school, thrusting our pelvises and squeezing our butts. We copied diets out of our own magazines and our mothers' magazines and followed them slavishly. We were pleased with ourselves if we ate only a frozen yogurt for lunch. We liked blond hair, popped collars, tanned skin, bony knees.

My mother allowed sugary carob Tiger's Milk bars as a treat because they whiffed of some ambiguous idea about health, but who even wanted to go to a health food store to get one? They smelled like bad breath and black mold, and the people who worked in them almost never looked good. *Wellness*, to the extent we'd heard of it, was for outliers, for the shell-shocked leftovers from hippie life, with their vans, their incense, their missing bras.

The super-entertaining *Road to Wellville*, a novel by T. C. Boyle that was published in 1993, is a fictionalized account of life at the Battle Creek Sanitarium in Michigan at the beginning of the twentieth century where the rich and miserable Eleanor Lightbody is subjected to lots of cold baths, electric shocks, and diets consisting exclusively of milk by the sinister Dr John Harvey Kellogg (who, in the film adaptation, was played by Anthony Hopkins post-*Silence of the Lambs*). Eleanor Lightbody is a caricature. She has more money than sense, a sadness deeper than the flesh, and so on, and embodies the traditional view of the wellness seeker: rich, female, it's-all-in-her-head. She finds true happiness and health only when the clinic burns down to the ground.

But even then, on the side, there was a growing hum of interest in the idea of something else, something more, some sort of extra health.

Holistic ideas about what it means to be well are not new inventions: these modes defined most medical practice until relatively recently. The practice of Ayurveda, which can be traced as far back as 3000 BC and which was eventually recorded in the Hindu sacred texts called the Vedas, is thought to be the earliest documented version of holistic approaches to health and Ayurvedic treatments, which are prescribed based on an individual's constitution (there are three main types, or doshas: vata, pitta, and kapha) and include nutritional advice and exercise. The guiding principle of Ayurveda is that the mind, body, and spirit are inextricably linked and that true health can be achieved only when all three are brought into balance. Ayurvedic practice was sought not only when disease presents; it was proposed as a way of life and, ideally, as a means of preventing disease from appearing in the first place.

Chinese medicine from the same period had a similar 'whole self' approach, treating the human as a miniature version of the universe, also placing an emphasis on balance by focusing on qi – a vital energy that flows through the whole body. Originally, it was believed that qi was thrown off when an ancestor had been dishonored; as thinking evolved, the focus came to be on finding harmony between the physical, emotional, and spiritual aspects of life.

In 400 BC, Hippocrates spent as much time considering prevention as he did cure. He eventually described disease as a product of diet, lifestyle, and environment, and as such, his treatments included a early version of art therapy, and he wrote on the benefits of deep tissue massage.

In many ways, early thinking about wellness in America was a way of reinventing the wheel: getting past the confines of Flexnerian medicine to theorize, like so many before us, that maybe there's more to health than the binaries of sick and not sick, disease and cure.

In the mid-1950s, a statistician named Dr Halbert L. Dunn delivered twenty-nine lectures at a Unitarian Universalist church in Arlington, Virginia, in which he defined high-level wellness as 'an integrated method of functioning which is oriented toward maximizing the potential of which the individual is capable. It requires that the individual maintain a continuum of balance and purposeful direction within the environment where he is functioning.' It's the 'purposeful direction' that intrigues. The proposal was that there was an option other than taking a reactive or even a passive relationship to health; even when you were feeling just fine, there was this other thing – this potentially better thing – to strive toward. Dunn wanted people to move away from striving only for the absence of disease and more toward an optimized state of 'high-level wellness.' He proposed that the 'state of being well is not a relatively flat, uninteresting area of "un-sickness." But is rather a fascinating and ever-changing panorama of life itself inviting exploration of its every dimension.' On the vast spectrum between health and its opposite (death), the individual can in fact exert a fair amount of control about where she lands.

The lectures attracted some attention, and Dunn published them as a book, *High-Level Wellness*, in 1961. Dr John Travis, the star of Dan Rather's report, bought Dunn's book on a clearance table at a bookstore for $2. ('Halbert Dunn [Hal] profoundly shaped my 46-year career,' Travis later said. 'His work led to my founding the first wellness center in the US in 1975. His death, the same week I opened the Center, might even be significant.')

But through the 1960s, these notions about self-care and alternative experimentation took root only in the counterculture.

Someone who found them there was Dr Andrew Weil. He trained at Harvard in the 1960s – during the reign of Timothy Leary and Richard Alpert. There he experimented with mescaline and psychedelics and published a graduate study on the effects of pot. After Weil received his medical degree in 1968 (against the objections of some more conservative senior Harvard faculty), he moved to San Francisco for an internship at a hospital that served the Haight. He then moved to Washington, D.C., for a two-year position with the National Institute of

Mental Health, but resigned after a year. The abrupt ending was, he says, because of 'his work on marijuana' during a time when 'the establishment view of the drug was as an unmitigated threat to mental health, more menacing than alcohol.'

Weil might have remained a fringe figure, like some red-eyed California hippies, but he liked mainstream culture, too. Friendly and avuncular and, crucially, medically credentialed, he has written books that advocate for plant-based diets, meditation, and exercise, reintroducing to the mainstream the notion that preventive care could be considered a form of medicine, too. Weil described strict adherence to evidence-based medicine as 'exactly analogous to religious fundamentalism.' His way forward had logic and rationality on its side: Why wouldn't you eat well, exercise, seek to nurture the whole self? His books *Eight Weeks to Optimum Health* and *The Healthy Kitchen* were both *New York Times* bestsellers.

In 1997, Weil appeared dramatically backlit on the cover of *Time* magazine, golden light pouring through the old-growth forest of his beard: 'Can This Guy Make You Healthy?' He looks like an enormous garden gnome, a balding Jerry Garcia. Weil might pose topless and smeared in mud, clutching a bouquet of fresh rosemary, and he was quite often high on some version of THC, but he was also a bona fide pioneer in bringing wellness ideas to the masses.

He was also one of the first to capitalize on the American wish to feel better. As much as changing the way we practice medicine in this country, Weil proved how much money there was to be made in the business of wellness. In studying Andrew Weil, we see how the model of a multichannel so-called lifestyle brand à la Ralph Lauren or Martha Stewart could work under an umbrella as big and as vague as 'health.' Weil has lent his name, endorsement, and image to vitamins, supplements, personal hygiene products, skin-care products ('mega-mushroom face serum' and so on), orthotics and footwear, medical devices, food prep equipment, and actual food, like 'savory country style salmon patties.' And he's made a whole lot of money doing it: as of 2019, Weil had donated $15 million for the construction of a new building for the Center for Integrative Medicine, which he had founded twenty-five years prior, at the University of Arizona. Naturally, the new building would bear his name.

The popularity of Andrew Weil presaged this new era: it's not just the rich or the Californians who are dissatisfied with traditional ideas about health. The current system of medicine in America has left a lot of people of all sorts of backgrounds feeling not very well and desperately seeking, and willing to spend money on, something new.

HOLISTIC, FUNCTIONAL, PROFITABLE

Andrew Weil brought wellness from the counterculture to the mainstream by backing a holistic gospel with a Harvard medical degree. That both/and approach, combining clinical standards with 'alternative' values, treatments, and aesthetics, has proven equally successful in today's premier incarnation of wellness-infused medicine: functional medicine.

Functional medicine is built on the notion that the principles proposed by Flexner – cleanliness, data gathering, evidence-based practice – might successfully merge with more ancient ideas about the worth of searching for the root causes of disease, as opposed to solely the cures. The idea for a systems-biology-based approach that focuses on identifying and addressing the root cause of disease was first described as functional medicine in 1990 by Dr Jeffrey Bland, a former professor of biochemistry at the University of Puget Sound in Tacoma, Washington, with a big interest in nutrition. Bland was never a practicing physician – his work veered in the direction of nutritional supplements – but his work marks an important moment in the idea of a more integrative approach to health care.

The emphasis that holistic traditions place on the body as a whole and on the practice of prevention is what advocates of the wellness movement say has been missing in an allopathic, solution-based system, and these traditions are often treated with reverence and with regret for what has been lost in the full-scale adoption of a modern system. That we might return to something more holistic is an almost-too-obvious prospect: of course we understand that health is complicated, of course we understand that the mind and the body and the immune system are all one, of course it makes sense that lifestyle plays a role in health outcomes. Why, Bland and others asked, was medical education not teaching about prevention, about nutrition, about alternative therapies that might not cure but have the potential to prevent?

Also, how was no one capitalizing on this great big market opportunity?

Proponents of functional medicine say that it holds the potential to change the way Americans think about health care. However true this is, the movement is certainly well suited to today's ever more profiteering medical industry, in which care is treated increasingly as a matter of choice, taste, political preference. Hospitals advertise on billboards, and, on TV, we can all recognize a commercial for a drug. Look at these attractive people thriving! This medical brand is most aligned with your other consumerist choices! This doctor is the Gap, but that one? That doctor might as well be Coco Chanel! We are consumers as much as we are patients (more than we are patients?).

In this landscape, a school of medicine that invites a bespoke combination of treatment approaches seems made to thrive. And indeed it has.

Once it was out there, the functional medicine mantle was taken up by a number of doctors, some of whom have become quite well known.

The dingy waiting room at Dr Frank Lipman's Eleven Eleven clinic on lower Fifth Avenue in Manhattan has held Maggie Gyllenhaal, Michelle Williams, Gwyneth Paltrow, Kevin Bacon, Sienna Miller, and others, all of whom appear on his testimonials page endorsing his work. 'I eat what he tells me to eat and drink what he tells me to drink and I feel great for it,' Gyllenhaal says. 'Frank… has solved every problem I've ever thrown his way,' says Williams. The actress Téa Leoni recommends one of his books: 'Can you imagine ONE pill that would clear up skin, bring calmness and clarity, make you happy and help prevent disease? [Dr Lipman's book] is as close as we'll ever get to that pill.'

Dr Lipman trained in South Africa, where he was born, and came to New York in 1984 as the chief medical resident at the Lincoln Medical Center in the Bronx, where he found himself increasingly drawn to the hospital's addiction center. It was the height of the crack epidemic, and the center was crowded with the miserable and the desperate. A program offering acupuncture to these patients fascinated Lipman: he suddenly saw his medical education as severely limited and set out to supplement what he knew with whatever else he could find, be it ancient or ignored or totally out there. Mostly, he thought, there had to be a way to focus on more than just the cure when treating a patient. He studied acupuncture, he experimented a lot, he wrote a number of books, like the bluntly titled *10 Reasons You Feel Old and Get Fat* and *Spent: End Exhaustion and Feel Great Again*. The books suggest that feeling old is not an inevitable by-product of aging but something easily avoided by paying attention. Paltrow endorsed his 2016 book, *Young and Slim for Life*, saying that by following Lipman's advice, one could travel through middle age with 'more vitality than a teenager.'

Knowing 'Frank' as Michelle Williams does is a big status signifier, an absolute insider flex. Lipman has hosted dinners with the celebrity chef David Bouley, and he is the chief medical officer of the glamorous, private, multi-city club the Well. While he admits to being a functional medicine doctor, he describes his practice, simply, as 'good medicine.' Eleven Eleven does not accept insurance.

Lipman is often practical; when I interviewed him in his office, I was red-eyed and sniffling from hay fever. We talked about the (widely disproven) theory of local honey as a hay fever cure; the Union Square farmers market a few blocks from Lipman's office was selling hyperlocal honey for exactly this reason. On the day I visited, the vendor was selling honey gathered from diverse locations, including 'Park Slope Rooftop,' 'Da Bronx,' and 'Washington Square Park' – Lipman was open to the idea of my giving it a go. But then he shrugged and told me to try Claritin, which was working well for his wife.

He is also avowedly open, often to things that feel mostly like common sense – that rest, water, sleep trifecta, for example. What is perhaps most intoxicating about his practice is his willingness to listen, the permission he gives to his patients to talk and explore and examine what they are feeling. He is a great giver of whole attention and a strong believer in the possibility of feeling great.

Another prominent figure in the functional medicine movement is Dr Mark Hyman, who is affiliated with the Cleveland Clinic's Center for Functional Medicine. (He also holds the title of chief medical officer at RoseBar at the Six Senses wellness resort in Ibiza.) Dr Hyman focuses a lot of his advice on eating better to age well, on the impact of the much-deployed term 'inflammation' on overall health. Hyman's often stated mission is to explore 'how five-thousand-year-old medicine can combine with twenty-first-century science to help you live longer,' and much of his method revolves around food. 'It seems that for many the cure for acne is at the end of their fork,' Hyman has said. He's also said, 'It's more important to understand the imbalances in your body's basic systems and restore balance, rather than name the disease and match the pill to the ill.'

Lipman and Hyman are peers, they are friends, and they share a commitment to fascia rolling, morning sun exposure, and a cold rinse at the end of a hot shower. They have spread their gospel through products and books and publicity and interviews while seeing only small numbers of patients.

It took a millennial to scale the idea of this kind of medicine, not just via books and supplements, but through in-person (or virtual) care given and received.

Enter Robin Berzin.

Dr. Berzin had a very traditional, very A-list medical education: she earned a summa cum laude undergraduate degree from the University of Pennsylvania and then went to medical school at Columbia University in New York. She took all the organic chemistry classes; she endured the chronic sleep deprivation of a residency in a big city hospital. She trailed from room to room clutching a coffee cup in a sea of other bright young people just like her, a mass of bobbing heads, a mass of shifting bodies in matching blue scrubs, listening to both attending doctors and the patients they serve.

This is the medical world that most of us can easily conjure from the other side: Chilly linoleum. Terrible lighting. Goose-pimpled skin emerging awkwardly from ripped paper gowns. The clunking sound of the medical scale, the stick and slip of the vinyl upholstery, the soft, backdated issues of *People* magazine. If you're in a city, the doctor's office is most likely up some stairs or an elevator. If you're in a smaller town, don't expect a plate glass window. Doctors' offices have historically been obscured from the traffic of mainstream life, with chilly, afterthought design. The entire experience suggests that a trip to the doctor is something to be endured rather than enjoyed, and, while it is imperative in getting *better* and in being *cured*, the remaining *being well* part is for elsewhere, something to consider in your own time. The conclusion of a doctor's appointment is usually met with a sense of relief. Back into your own soft clothing, back into the better light. The writer Meghan O'Rourke has spent a lot of time in doctors' offices, both as a patient herself and as a companion to her mother, who had cancer. She writes: 'I was startled by the profound discomfort I felt, especially in hospitals. Doctors at times seemed brusque and even hostile toward us. The lighting was harsh, the food terrible, the rooms loud and devoid of comfort. Were people there to heal? This did not appear to matter.'

While Berzin was training to become a doctor, she was also becoming a yogi. And she was also realizing, in her clinical practice, how absent preventive health measures (nutrition, for example) were from what she was learning in school. While working at a walk-in clinic, she realized that just instructing her patients to give up soda could make a big improvement in their health. If she could do so much with one such minor intervention, what could she do if she had more time to understand the circumstances and routines of her patients' lives?

Eventually, she found herself attracted to functional medicine, as Drs. Lipman and Hyman had been before her. She liked the logic of it all; she was intrigued by how the things she had learned outside school – as a yoga teacher, for example – informed what she learned inside school and saw infinite ways to blend the two.

'We designed a system for saving your life, not a system for helping you live,' she told me, hence her desire to find a potentially better idea. Basically, if you're going to get in a car crash and break all your bones, you'd better hope to land in a great big modern Western hospital as fast as you can. But if you want to avoid the whole crash in the first place, or if you want to heal fully once you've been pasted back into shape, how would you go about that?

For Berzin, this was an important realization. 'That's it,' she told her husband, 'I'm going to be a hippie doctor.'

While Drs. Lipman and Hyman tend to treat small numbers of patients at considerable cost, Berzin is attempting to merge the concept of functional, integrative medicine with big VC capital. The company she founded is Parsley Health, and it has, to date, raised more than $100 million for its membership-model, multi-city GP practice offices whose New York City flagship was written up in *Vogue*. ('Upon entry, Parsley Health's light-filled Manhattan space feels more like a trendy café or a millennial members-only club than a doctors' office. Air-purifying plants line the walls, and a custom essential oil blend of lemon, basil, and cedarwood wafts through every room. The seating is mid-century modern, and the kitchen is stocked with Devoción coffee, Three Pigs tea, and Pilot kombucha on tap.') Berzin understands that medicine is increasingly a retail prospect and that plenty of people feel the way that O'Rourke does about the experience of seeking care. A Los Angeles center is similarly well designed, with floor-to-ceiling windows and, according to *Architectural Digest*, 'a mindful balance of neutral hues.' It looks like somewhere you'd go with a group of girl-friends for brunch, as if it could happily host a bridal shower for Kate Hudson and a bunch of her pretty friends. 'We paid close attention to the color palette to instill a sense of calm, activating a parasympathetic state,' Hilary Koyfman, the interior designer, told *Architectural Digest*, specifying that some of the colors used are Benjamin Moore's Soft Chinchilla and Monticello Rose.

One of Berzin's top selling points is this: the average American spends nineteen minutes a year in conversation with a primary care doctor; the average member at Parsley spends two hundred, and, if she has her way, she will have more and more doctors seeing more and more patients this way. Parsley announced in 2023 that it is now considered an in-network primary care provider for more than ten million potential patients in New York and California.

A Parsley membership begins with an extensive series of inquiries and tests that suggest, in their very thoroughness, that the patient is to be heard, that the patient will be believed.

No clue is too silly, no idea too small. How often in your life have you taken antibiotics? How was your dental hygiene as a kid? What do you eat every day, how are your friendships, do you work out, do you recover, what worries you when you wake up in the night, and how often do you do that? The new vocabulary of wellness weaves in, out, and around the whole operation – what is happening in your microbiome, where does your inflammation lurk? Do you have *brain fog*? How many supplements are you willing to take?

The legitimizing of discomfort may well be Parsley's biggest innovation: at Parsley, you are invited to reveal what ails you, in as much detail as you can, and you are also invited to name problems not typically considered serious and to embark on a journey into how to improve them. As Berzin once posted on her highly active Instagram account, 'Even in a perfect storm you can enjoy watching the weather.'

But it's more than just the listening. This new way of going to the doctor feels specifically targeted at women in just the same way that fashion is: Am I at the doctor? Am I in a spa? Am I actually just *inside* Instagram? At Parsley, I consulted with a doctor over a lovely, veined Carrara marble tabletop while sitting on a nicely upholstered banquette. Under the warm yellow lighting, my skin didn't even look blue. No one left me alone to shiver in a paper robe; no one made me stand on a cruel, wobbly scale. Parsley members are invited to use the lobby, with its low sapphire-blue sofa and soft Berber rugs, with its north- and west-facing loft-style windows and original pressed-tin ceiling, as a gathering place and a respite, whether you have an appointment that day or not.

An executive at Parsley Health told me that the office design is in fact 'biophilic,' which is a philosophy that posits that built spaces should promote healing and that this kind of healing is best facilitated by simulating a connection to nature inside a built space. In biophilic design, the indoor/nature connection should be visual as well as non-visual (as in plants that you can both see *and* smell), and airflow and light should be as consistent with the natural environment as possible, so no glaring LEDs or air conditioners turned to blast. A nice view and a little gurgling water element are ideal. Both the Hanging Gardens of Babylon and Frank Lloyd Wright's Fallingwater are often cited as triumphs of biophilic design. The tenets, as defined by the sustainability consulting firm Terrapin Bright Green, include the following:

> *Refuge:* 'a place for withdrawal from environmental conditions or the main flow of activity, in which the individual is protected from behind and overhead';
> *Risk/peril:* 'an identifiable threat coupled with a reliable safeguard.'

It's a perfect moment for medicine to start looking good: as retail migrates further and further online, storefronts and strip malls find themselves desperately in search of new tenants and life. Will future generations even know that toilet paper and flour and snow boots were ever available right down the street? The suburban shopping mall began its death spiral even as it ascended: when the Mall of America debuted, the Minneapolis megalopolis with an enormous, anchoring Sears, it was unimaginable what Amazon – then a small idea in a Seattle garage – would bring, that the mini golf, the aquarium, and the Hooters would be more important to the mall's survival than the gigantic Abercrombie & Fitch.

Each year the percentage of retail transactions in the United States that takes place online increases significantly, with no slowdown in sight. A 2016 Pew Research survey found 80 percent of Americans had shopped online – the 20 percent who hadn't tend to be older – and a 2022 Raydiant study of consumer habits found that a majority of respondents *prefer* to shop online.

How To Be Well

For years the central retail street of my Brooklyn neighborhood was in grim shape: at its lowest point, around 20 percent of its storefronts were empty, while UPS clogged traffic on the narrow blocks, disgorging mountains of boxes to doorsteps and stoops. When the scaffold came down around an inviting, earth-toney place called Oula, a lot of people spent a lot of time looking in the windows, hoping that maybe it was a friendly bookshop, a place to get a cup of tea? But it was an ob-gyn practice with an emphasis on fertility and childbirth, a place that might offer 'refuge' from the 'risk and peril' outside its doors. Oula was more elegantly designed than the two urgent care offices that opened on the same street, and the family dentistry practice was somewhere in between: not quite so Pinterest, but not traditionally clinical in appearance, either. Several blocks away is an outpost of Tend, a nicely designed dental practice chain with the tagline 'Care at Tend isn't just painless, it's a pleasure.' The dentist! A pleasure?

The street-level retail trade in the part of Brooklyn where I live is now concentrated on health above all else: there is not a butcher on Montague Street, but if you want to have your blood pressure checked, or your throat swabbed, or a wart removed, you have choices. The ten-minute walk from my house to my children's school takes me past at least four businesses offering to solve a long roster of illnesses and discomforts through the use of medical marijuana and CBD. Their lobbies are always so welcoming: upholstered seating, potted plants, gummies and pills and books carefully styled on open wooden shelving beside organically shaped, neutral-toned pottery and old-school Edison light.

So many of these environments share a certain High Wellness/2000s boutique hotel lobby aesthetic. It's a look that feels like refuge for burnt-out digital natives who have some vague collective longing for a 1970s-ish aesthetic – not as the 1970s were lived, but as they are now experienced via photographs leached of strong pigment by both technology and time. I once interviewed an artist who told me about coming across old photographs of Woodstock: Do you see how everyone was beautiful, she asked, beautiful and thin? I did see it because she was right. They were all beautiful, with shiny hair and clear skin and flat stomachs. 'It's because they did not have preservatives in their food yet,' she told me, 'it's because their marijuana was organically grown.' Wellness nostalgia, from before it was even a thing. A yearning for weak 'organic' pot grown on windowsills and in secret gardens rather than on organized, regulated farms.

These spaces can feel like a deliberate blurring of spaces designated frivolous – spas, salons, matcha cafés – and medical, which is exactly where so much wellness lives. Modern Age, a now-closed company founded by a former Amazon executive, tested and prescribed hormone treatments *and* Botox. Trellis was an egg-freezing clinic that served celery juice and kept gut-friendly, probiotic-dense kombucha on tap. (Trellis listed as its attributes an 'Insta-worthy studio with phone chargers, a juice bar and a modern workspace, we want you to feel inspired during the egg freezing journey. Meet with our fertility nutritionists anytime or bring a friend to enjoy a juice.' That office had metallic wallpaper printed with an inspirational quotation by Michelle Obama and a weekly delivery of Juliet roses.)

Part of the idea is that one shouldn't expect to become better in a space that feels artificial or cold. Anything obviously synthetic in form or material is not wellness; materials must be natural in origin and as close to whole in presentation as possible. Colors should not pop or distract or assault the senses, just as furniture should not have edges that could batter the shins. The wish, in these spaces, is for clarity and simplicity, for safety, for a nontoxic, underwhelming space where one is soothed, cocooned, buttressed from the corrupt and toxified world.

It is a profoundly feminine idea about care: these spaces use the established visual vernacular of the trendy fashion boutique, which has historically been designed to attract women. They have the same ship-lap wood paneling, the same woven hangings on the wall, the same fair-trade baskets sprinkled here and there, the same pretty colors on the walls. That the environments are so aesthetically like fashion boutiques suggests that these are spaces in which women are welcome and might finally be considered first, but it also furthers the notion that for women good health is a luxury, that good health is for *sale*, that good health can be pursued like a hobby, like fun. The experience of paying to achieve an alternative, better you is not unlike the experience of buying a new pair of shoes or a very expensive bag. In this case, though, you are the product, so long as you can afford to buy yourself back.

Because these environments are so familiar to women, it can take a moment to realize how bizarre it can be to occupy such an overtly patient/customer hybrid position. This is not beside the point; it is the point. There is just so much stuff to buy! When I first joined Parsley, I was sent for a blood draw that involved fourteen vials of blood, several plastic vials of spit, and a beaker of urine. I was also given a $125 vitamin B_{12} shot on the spot and then sold a series of Parsley-branded supplements – vitamin D_3, magnesium glycinate for sleep, and a protein meal-replacement powder that the Parsley doctor suggested in place of my typical breakfast of organic kefir made from the milk of local cows that, I was assured, led uncommonly joyful lives.

Although I had been conditioned by wellness literature to carefully consider the origins of everything I put into my body, to always choose a 'whole' food rather than something processed, this flavored powder was sold to me as a superior option.

Alternative doctors often criticize Big Medicine for being in bed with doctors, and the evidence is certainly there (Purdue

Holistic, Functional, Profitable

Pharma and the opioid epidemic come to mind) to back them up. What they are less comfortable addressing is the parallel system they have created with their proprietary lines of tablets, lavender eye cushions, and protein shakes. Often, differences have more to do with scarcity than with nutrition: Why do we consider almond or cashew butter more 'well' than the peanut butter of our childhoods? Why is acai a wellness berry in a way that blueberries and strawberries are not? Acai is a small purple berry that grows in Central and South American rain forests, is similarly high in antioxidants to other, more common-in-the-U.S. berries, but an 'acai bowls!' sign is a message that an establishment has converted to 'wellness.' (Seldom mentioned is the bitterness of the berry, which means common preparations are typically loaded with sugar.)

I have noticed, over time, a shift in Berzin's own positioning. In the early days of Parsley her online presence felt more traditionally medical: she played up her MD bona fides, often posting safe ideas like 'Fast food is making us sick. Fast medicine is keeping us sick,' and 'Sugar is a core driver of every major illness: diabetes, cancer, PCOS, heart disease, autoimmune disease, and depression.'

But it was also evolving into the fuzzier territories of manifestation and abundance and gratitude: 'The more peaceful I am the more abundance comes into my life.' That sort of thing. Jade rollers turned up.

Berzin documents life with three children. She admits that it is difficult but does not mention if a tantrum happened after she told her toddler that she'd have to throw out her Easter candy save one very small piece. It's an appealing strategy, and many of the questions in her comments section are about where she got that lovely top, the one that shows that even a hardworking mother of three can achieve a tight set of washboard abs. In 2023, she documented a 'life-changing' trip to Burning Man.

Her mission to create well women was only bolstered by her success in herself becoming one of the highest degree.

Parsley is finding its niche more and more crowded: there's Tia, which was founded by Carolyn Witte and Felicity Yost. Witte, the CEO, describes herself as a 'brand and design enthusiast – a by-product of her time at Google's Creative Lab,' and Yost, who oversees product, marketing, finance, and operations, describes herself as a 'data enthusiast with a deep passion for health and wellness.' Neither woman is a doctor, but both women have often been patients and approach the project from that perspective. Tia's mission is to offer a range of services considered women's health care in a single, beautifully designed setting (eight brick-and-mortar locations are in New York, California, and Arizona, with more to come) or online. Tia clinics offer ob-gyn services, primary care, mental health professionals, acupuncturists, and pelvic floor therapy all in bright, poppy spaces designed by Alda Ly, who is the same architect who worked on Parsley. 'It was important to Tia that we create a space that patients are drawn to so that they're more encouraged to stay on top of their health,' Ly said to *Healthcare Design* magazine. 'We're not small men,' Allie Ball, Tia's vice president of creative, added, 'yet a lot of healthcare practices have been designed or treated us like such. At Tia, we try to do the opposite and think about what a woman would want to feel comfortable in their experience.'

Liv by Advantia Health, another company that says it is 'women's healthcare, reimagined,' also hired Ly to design its flagship location in Washington, D.C. 'Designed for your comfort and convenience,' the Liv website reads, 'our calming space makes prioritizing women's health and wellness an enjoyable experience.'

An overwhelming majority of entrepreneurs who work in functional medicine (and functional-medicine-adjacent businesses) are highly successful women pursuing their second career. Many are refugees from high-pressure, image-conscious industries, like entertainment, or fashion, or finance, with punishing hours and an absence of work-life balance. They'd all experienced some version of what we now call burnout, which took the shape of hives, or back problems, or skin problems, or bloat, and had been cured by the discovery of some protocol and gone evangelical, eager to share the tools of their miraculous transformation with the world. Rebecca Parekh, a cofounder and CEO of the Well, for example, worked at the trading desk of a bank; on her first vacation in five years, she found herself paralyzed with anxiety and a crooked back. She next sought employment with the New Age guru Deepak Chopra, and it was from there that she got the idea to establish the Well.

The author of an exhaustive guide to 'detox' got into it while pregnant, when she'd spend all day working at an investment management firm and all night researching safe synthetic nipples and weeping with anxiety over the threats of mattress off-gassing and BPAs. The venture capitalist behind some of the industry's biggest names quit her job in banking when her hands were too covered in sores to show off her engagement ring. She identified gluten as the culprit and set out to angel invest in female-founded companies that could help women feel better.

Meghan Markle's first post-Megxit business endeavors involved investing in Clevr Blends, a 'women-led, mission-driven wellness company' that markets powdered matcha and a variety of 'superlattes and superteas.' Arianna Huffington sold her namesake website (*The Huffington Post*) a few years after passing out with exhaustion and breaking her cheekbone – an incident she calls 'my blessing' – and in 2016 founded a company called Thrive, which brings wellness to corporations and runs a sideline in the promotion, and the accessorizing, of sleep. Chelsea Clinton is an investor in Oula Health.

None of these women has ditched a well-compensated life, however, for an ascetic vow: the idea that pursuing wellness can be every bit as lucrative as what they've left behind is crucial. As Witte said, 'My favorite topic: building a mission-driven business that puts women in the driver's seat in the exam room *and* in the boardroom. Yes, it's all connected!'

In my own circles, I was surprised to learn that Sabine Heller, a woman I used to see around the fashion world, was unwell. She had both endometriosis and something called CIU that she says stands for 'Nobody knows why I have sudden extreme facial swelling and a rash the color of pomegranate!' Heller no longer produces parties and runway shows: she is instead working at Sollis Health, among the Chuck Close paintings and copies of *The Paris Review* that are scattered with artist monographs in the waiting room. Her new offices, which serve tea made by the legendary scenester and Wes Anderson muse Waris Ahluwalia, are not hugely different looking from those she'd inhabited in the worlds of fashion and design.

Sollis was conceived quietly in 2016 by Dr Bernard Kruger, an internist who has long ogled the tonsils and inner ears of Bono, Sting, Ben Stiller, and Ralph Lauren (among others) on Manhattan's Upper East Side. His son, Ben Kruger, is Sollis's cofounder, and he's proud of their fancy offices. 'The thoughtfulness that goes into curating art reflects the thoughtfulness and attention to detail that goes into the individualized medical care we provide to our members,' Ben told *Forbes* magazine. It was gathering steam – often in partnership with luxury real estate, like the ur-private social club San Vicente Bungalows in Los Angeles, which offered early discounts on Sollis to its members and guests – but it really took off as a concept during COVID, when tests and vaccines were often hard to come by and it had become normal to wait in a line for hours in order to board a flight or visit your mom. Easy testing and, when it was available, access to treatment were the ultimate luxuries in that shakiest of times.

Therein lies the double edge of functional medicine as it mostly exists today. It can be a perfect marriage of mainstream medical treatment, holistic practice, and thoughtfully designed setting, but it's usually offered only at a deeply exclusionary price point, and it often improves access for a population whose access is not terrible to begin with.

And for those who had to wait in line for COVID vaccines, there are still plenty of ways to access wisdom (and chic design) at the intersection of medicine and wellness. They are everywhere! The only caveat is that many of the available gurus aren't exactly board certified.

KOOKS

There's a certain amount of openness required to venture into the world of alternative medicines, a certain amount of willingness – or desperation – to accept evidence of the sort we have been taught not to value. When it works, it's wonderful. But it does make an alarming amount of space for the kooks and the quacks and the snake oil to slip in. In the process of being told that so much we take as a given is, if not wrong, then at least flawed, we can find it difficult to parse the rest.

Aubrey Gordon and Michael Hobbes's fantastic podcast, *Maintenance Phase*, provides a stringent and highly entertaining debunking of many of wellness's most famous showmen. One of my favorite episodes dismantles Bragg's apple cider vinegar (ACV), a weird supermarket product I have spent months adding to glasses of water because of an endlessly repeated wellness theory that it can fix... everything. The story of Bragg's, though, is a perfect case study in how these myths are built and how they endure. It starts with Johnny Appleseed, of all people, who it turns out was a real person named John Chapman, but he was not exactly the adorable folk hero of our collective imagination; he was a Swedenborgian Christian missionary who came of age during the Industrial Revolution in America, a moment when there existed a lot of fear and anxiety about modernization. Chapman thought that the common method of planting apple trees – known as grafting – was alarming and, according to his belief system, cruel to the apples. His mission was to plant apple trees the biblical way – seeding – which made for sour, fibrous, gnarly apples that were best used in fermentation, yielding big supplies of both alcoholic cider and vinegar.

Here is where Chapman's story intersects with the story of Paul Bragg, one of America's earliest wellness pioneers, who, it turns out, is a liar nearly on the scale of George Santos. Bragg claimed he was born on a farm in Virginia in 1881, and he claimed that he was diagnosed with tuberculosis at sixteen, which he cured with some clean living at a Swiss clinic, and then he claimed that he was an Olympic wrestler. And so on.

He launched what he called the Bragg Health Crusade tour in 1929, sharing these and other stories about himself and lecturing about the benefits of fasting and the benefits of apple cider vinegar. His lectures have been cited as influential by the founders of GNC, Gardenburger, and Dr Scholl's.

Except that many of his health claims, and the life story he told, including his birthplace and birth date, were false. When he died in 1976, he left the company to his daughter Patricia Bragg, except it turns out she wasn't really his daughter; she was his ex-daughter-in-law. The American Medical Association called him a 'food faddist,' and the postmaster general issued a fraud order against him and his company.

'This was part of an American folk healing tradition,' Gordon says on her podcast. 'He offered people the sense that what they had already been doing was a really good thing to do, not just for their own health, but for their own virtue and character because of this sort of deeply Christian language that [the Braggs] use. It's not just a matter of caring for your body; it's a matter of your piety and your ability to resist temptation… He's doing a thing that happens still, which is getting very comfortable muddling up people's perceived health with their character and morality and worth as people. All of that is getting dumped into the same bucket.'

Listening to Gordon, one would assume that Bragg's company went out of business during an age of readily accessible information, an age when it's easy to learn that there is no evidence connecting apple cider vinegar to improved health, but that's not what happened at all. Instead, Bragg's just kept claiming what it always had, and then a chance encounter with celebrity took care of the rest.

Orlando Bloom and Katy Perry bought the company with a private equity firm in 2019 – Patricia Bragg was a parishioner at the church where Perry's parents were pastors, and she was about to retire – and went on to promote the hell out of it. On *Jimmy Fallon*, Bloom told the story of falling in love with Perry over vinegar water. 'We both had bottles of apple cider vinegar,' he says, 'and I was like, this is it!' The Well+Good wellness platform recommends it for curing everything from constipation to pimples. ACV is now widely available as a supplement in tablet and gummy form for people who don't like the taste (one favorite of mine for its name alone is Swolverine ACV Gummies).

Debunking, it seems, has no effect on the popularity of a remedy if the claims are grand enough. In fact, it can have the opposite effect; it can elevate the method or substance in question to the status of a true *secret*.

'Is Gwyneth Paltrow wrong about everything?' asks the title of a book by a Canadian public health scholar named Timothy Caulfield. A cottage industry has sprung up around the debunking of Goop, largely because we seem to keep getting suckered in.

Goop has a history of promoting alternative healers, using the popular platform to amplify their techniques. Goop answers with an innocent 'just asking questions!' stance, but it presents a danger far more real than the shameless attention grabs. Jennifer Gunter, a San Francisco gynecologist, has become famous for dissembling the myths Goop pushed via her blog *Wielding the Lasso of Truth*, and later on a Substack called *The Vajenda*.

It started with a response she published in 2015 to Paltrow's recommending vaginal steaming to balance female hormone levels. 'It's one of the core beliefs of patriarchy. That women are dirty inside,' Gunter wrote. 'And yet Goop presents this as female empowerment?... It's bad feminism. And it's bad science.' She took Goop on for a number of disproven theories: about underwire bras causing breast cancer, about the benefits of coffee enemas. 'Dear God, no,' Gunter wrote in her book *The Vagina Bible*. 'I. Just. Can't. Even.'

Caulfield, for his part, argues that Paltrow is perhaps not the best messenger for ideas about beauty and health. 'The fact that individuals who have won the beauty-gene lottery are setting universal beauty standards is a bit like using NBA power forwards to inspire people to endeavor to be tall.'

If you want to get really mad, just listen to Paltrow's 2019 interview with Caroline Myss, a self-described medical intuitive who is also a 'deep believer in the power of prayer.' In a decidedly un-Flexnerian way, Myss's evidence is all anecdotal. She knew she was an intuitive because a colleague once said to her, 'My neighbor isn't feeling well,' and Myss replied, 'She has leukemia.' Myss also says, 'My skill is that I have a natural ability to sense what's wrong, and it's directed towards your health. And everybody has that ability. Your body's system is naturally directed to tell you what is wrong in order to keep you alive... I have an ability to read yours as well as you can read your own.'

When Paltrow asks her what advice to give to a friend with chronic bladder infections that don't respond to antibiotics, Myss says, 'This is one of those jewels you can take with you for the rest of your life forever: You are like a ship and a ship always will go back to balance... When anything goes wrong in your body or in your life, imagine that it's trying to get back to balance. So instead of looking at the bladder, first thing you should ask is, what's out of balance and go at it that way. How am I acting in relationships? Is there a struggle, what am I worried about, and how am I handling those patterns? If you are in anguish about something and you are repeating your anguish to people without actually resolving it, that's a type of poison that can get into your bladder.'

'So we are responsible for getting to deeper levers of feeling accountability ourselves?' Paltrow asks.

'There's always something you can resolve or do in some way,' Myss says. 'Yes.'

A difficult message to deliver, I would imagine, to a patient with terminal cancer, or any other horrible, terminal disease.

Showmen promising miracle cures have been putting on shows forever. In fourteenth-century Europe medical 'professionals' used to pitch tents in small villages and towns to 'cure' people of their ills – blindness, limps, and so on – using expensive potions that historians now understand to have been various combinations of alcohol and narcotics. The practice continued until relatively recently: in nineteenth-century America, the medications sold by these traveling salesmen/entertainers were called patent medicines, and they had names like Hamlin's Wizard Oil and Kickapoo Indian Oil. Cocaine was a common additive, and celebrities were popular endorsers. There was even a 1932 animated short film called *Betty Boop, M.D.*, in which Betty persuades a whole town to buy her mysterious health tonic, Jippo, which is really just water from a hydrant. But it makes a baby grow into a... man-sized baby. And so on.

Medicine road shows have long been outlawed, but it might be difficult to locate the differences between them and, say, the Goop traveling wellness road shows, where my $1,000 ticket bought access not only to Paltrow's infuriating onstage conversation with Caroline Myss but also to a session with a psychic/middle school English teacher from Long Island who told me to listen to the voices in my head, and some itchy, acupuncture-ish 'crystal ear seeds' that I stopped trying to pick out only once the early-evening vodka cart appeared. (Mixers were of the fresh fruit variety. Jippo, indeed!) Some of the advice was almost comic, if harmless. I watched a woman in a full G. Label Goop-branded outfit take assiduous notes in a Goop-branded notebook throughout the psychic/English teacher's lecture and then raise her hand.

'I keep seeing the same number everywhere I go,' she said. 'This one number just keeps coming up. What does it mean?'

'It means,' the English teacher said, 'it means you're on exactly the right path.' The woman looked so comforted: her shoulders settled a bit in her puff-sleeved top. She had gotten the assurance she craved, which maybe was worth the price of admission.

But then I was subjected to a session with a psychic 'medium' who claimed to contact a recently deceased friend – a disturbing and upsetting experience that I recounted to a journalist friend on the street the next morning. She immediately referred me to a recently published *New York Times Magazine* article about the Guerrilla Skeptics – a group of no-nonsense Northern California volunteers turned off by the way that so-called psychics and mediums have been using social media to con people into believing they have a connection with the afterlife or the great beyond, when really they just have strong Wi-Fi.

'He's okay with how he died,' the 'medium' told me that day, as all the lucky women with their blowouts and their leggings stared. 'It will help others. He is at peace.' I was outraged after the experience. I called Susan Gerbic, the founder of the Guerrilla Skeptics and a fellow of the Committee for Skeptical Inquiry, and told her what had happened. She was able to find all of the information the 'medium' had relayed in just a few short moments on Google. An obvious trick, I suppose, but in this case I found efforts to reassure me to be an offense rather than a comfort.

I wasn't sure, in the days that followed, if what I had done was fair. I was, after all, there as a journalist, not a genuine seeker, and perhaps a true seeker would have found comfort, would have overlooked the method. Perhaps seekers have done so forever in search of solace. Was I annoyed that I hadn't been left to observe in peace? The woman before me had been told that her grandmother thought she should go ahead with her kitchen renovation, and she visibly exhaled; that all seemed fine to me, safe. Know your lane, wellness! I wanted to shout. Kitchen renovations, sure. But please don't try to go deeper. Not in public, not for me.

The Oprah Winfrey Show hosted a medical road show for years, bringing its viewers an assemblage of doctors and healers and psychics and friends. Some of the theories and solutions they promoted were more plausible than others.

In the early days of Winfrey's career as a talk show host, one of her big draws was her willingness to 'go there' on just about any stigmatized topic. She spoke frankly and openly about depression, alcoholism, child abuse (her own included), and incest. In a then-rare moment of candor for a woman in the public eye, she was honest about how hard it was to stay thin: in 1988, Winfrey wheeled sixty-seven pounds of fat in a Radio Flyer red wagon onto the set of her show to demonstrate how much she had lost on a new diet.

At a certain point, Winfrey decided that it wasn't enough to just publicly name suffering; it was also time to heal. In an interview with the writer Bill Adler in 1994, she said, 'The time has come for this genre of talk shows to move on from dysfunctional whining and complaining and blaming. I have had enough of people's dysfunction. I don't want to spend an hour listening to somebody blaming their mother. So to say that I am tired – yes I am. I'm tired of it. I think it's completely unnecessary. We're all aware that we do have some problems and we need to work on them. What are you willing to do about it? And that is what our shows are going to be about.' In 2000, Winfrey launched O, The Oprah Magazine with the mission 'to help women see every experience and challenge as an opportunity to grow and discover their best self. To convince women that the real goal is becoming more of who they really are.'

Oprah also assembled her own medical board, which had no problem challenging the medical hegemony and encouraging her viewers to question it, too. In 2012, Oprah traveled to Brazil for a special episode on an illiterate faith healer and 'psychic surgeon' called John of God, who performed a surgery on a woman with a paralyzed arm. As he made an incision above the woman's breast, Oprah says, 'I didn't know if I was going to throw up or have diarrhea on camera.' Later, she interviews John of God beneath a mango tree and tells him she was 'humbled by the experience,' and then asks him 'what color' cancer is when he identifies it. John of God was later arrested for sexually abusing his patients, with his accusers detailing rapes in which he claimed to be transferring 'cleansing energy' from his body into theirs. He has been sentenced to spend the rest of his life in prison.

One of the most meta-medical conversations to ever happen on *The Oprah Winfrey Show* took place in 2007 when Winfrey invited the actress Jenny McCarthy on the show. McCarthy's son had been diagnosed with autism, and McCarthy believed both that the autism was the direct result of vaccinations and that the condition was reversible. The conversation went like this:

McCarthy: First thing I did – Google. I put in autism and I started my research.

Oprah: Thank God for Google.

McCarthy: I'm telling you!

Oprah: Thank God for Google.

McCarthy: The University of Google is where I got my degree from… and I put in autism and something came up that changed my life, that led me on this road to recovery, which said autism – it was in the corner of the screen – is reversible and treatable. And I said, what? That has to be an ad for a hocus-pocus thing, because if autism is reversible and treatable, well, then it would be on *Oprah*.

The audience roared. Because it was on *Oprah*, the mountains of evidence against the vaccine-autism causation didn't matter; it was suddenly plausible. The walls between patients and medicine had collapsed: the perception that mainstream science was infinitely fallible at best and dangerously negligent at worst had been validated by one of the most popular and admired women in the country.

This kind of full-throated enthusiasm for pseudo-medical claims on *Oprah* created at least one serious star who would go on to mold mainstream ideas about how to be well: Dr Oz spun off with his own show in 2009, and at the height of COVID in 2020 he was reaching 22 million viewers, according to the Annenberg Public Policy Center at the University of Pennsylvania, and had ten Daytime Emmy Awards. He'd also published a dozen books, founded *The Good Life* magazine, and trademarked the phrase 'America's Doctor,' which Winfrey first called him in 2004. Like the traveling medicine men who preceded him, Dr Oz is a showman with a tendency to make over-the-top promises and to use spectacular props, like two human hearts (one thriving, one not), or an empty colon, which looked like a blanched mushroom. Once, during a segment about acne, Oz popped a massive foam pimple, which spouted coconut cream. The information shared on his show is very hit-or-miss: Oz holds several patents for methods and devices used in lifesaving heart surgeries and transplants, but he has also been hauled in front of Congress for telling his audience about a 'miraculous' (and entirely bogus) green coffee pill that could make anyone lose weight. On that episode his star guest was described as a 'naturopathic doctor,' but he was in fact a marketing executive representing companies that sold green coffee extract. Oz often uses words like 'magic' and 'miracle' in his descriptions of understudied practices, so it's not entirely surprising that in 2014 the *British Medical Journal* concluded, following an extensive review, that *at least* 50 percent of the advice given on his show during the previous year was not backed by scientific evidence or was contradicted by publicly available data, and many of the bits that were deemed legitimate were hardly groundbreaking – 'don't smoke,' for example.

Oz's politics predate his 2022 run for Senate: his conservative leanings have revealed themselves for years. There was the episode about gay conversion therapy – which aired in 2012 but would later be scrubbed from his website – and in 2016, following a softball interview and a hands-off 'exam' with the then presidential candidate Donald Trump, who had been under fire for producing a patently false doctor's note, Oz declared Trump, who would later endorse Oz's candidacy for the Senate, in good health.

In 2015, a group of medical doctors and professors cosigned a letter to Columbia University, where Oz still taught, that read: 'Dr. Oz has repeatedly shown disdain for science and for evidence-based medicine... Worst of all, he has manifested an egregious lack of integrity by promoting quack treatments and cures in the interest of personal financial gain. Thus, Dr Oz is guilty of either outrageous conflicts of interest or flawed judgements about what constitutes appropriate medical treatments, or both. Whatever the nature of his pathology, members of the public are being misled and endangered.' Oz, who was once described by the dean of the faculty of Columbia as one of the most talented surgeons he had ever met, was relieved of his position at Columbia during his Senate campaign. It was one thing for Oz to bring Reiki practitioners into the operating theater (as he'd been known to do) – at worst it would be a menace – but it was another thing for him to profit so baldly off information so easily proven dangerous or even just wrong.

In a country where the average doctor's visit lasts around fifteen minutes, where the number of Americans with an ongoing and consistent relationship with a GP declines each year, lots of people know Oz and his trim blue scrubs better than they know any other MD. He looks quite healthy himself, he is famous, *he is on TV.* If you can't afford a trip to Parsley, who then is listening? GP, after all, are also the initials of the founder of Goop.

During the spring of 2023, I got to watch a medical conversation morph into a wellness road show in real time. I had written an article for *The New York Times* in December 2022 about the race to monetize menopause: the formerly unmentionable category had become lucrative. A number of high-profile celebrities (ranging from Oprah herself to Michelle Obama to Drew Barrymore and Naomi Watts) were willing to publicly address their own midlife changes. When Anne Fulenwider, whom I knew from her time as editor in chief of *Marie Claire* magazine, went in search of funding for Alloy, her telehealth menopause company, she met a male investor then under thirty who leaped at the chance. 'I've been looking for a menopause company!' he told her.

Everything was lining up beautifully: A legitimate hole in the marketplace had been created by decades of neglect. Medical practitioners received a shockingly small amount of training in the treatment of symptoms associated with menopause; a 2013 Johns Hopkins survey of ob-gyn residents found that less than one in five had received any formal training in menopause medicine.

Also, ideas about the safety of hormone replacement therapy (HRT) were changing. Beginning in the early 1990s, a $625 million effort known as the Women's Health Initiative undertook a decade-long study of 16,600 diverse women in an effort to evaluate the relative efficacy and dangers of HRT. The results, published in 2002, reported that HRT use in postmenopausal women increased the risk for a number of frightening conditions, including breast cancer, heart disease, and blood clots. Usage of HRT immediately dropped, with insurance claims declining 30 percent in the first six months after the study was published. By 2009, these were down more than 70 percent. The number of American women using HRT stayed low for the next decade.

But more recent research suggests that the results of this study were at worst flawed and at best misrepresented in most media coverage. HRT could in fact be both safe and effective for a range of women experiencing unpleasant menopausal symptoms, like brain fog and painful sex and hot flashes. In July 2022, the North American Menopause Society (NAMS) published a new position, stating that instead of broad restrictions the risks and benefits of HRT should be addressed individually between doctors and patients. A few weeks after I published my article, *The New York Times Magazine* published a piece by the writer Susan Dominus; she was one of many women who had taken the new advice and was finding tremendous relief with HRT. 'Women Have Been Misled About Menopause,' went the headline.

The new NAMS position paper came out as the pandemic was petering out, right when the public's willingness to be treated virtually had accelerated tremendously, almost entirely because of need. The idea of being prescribed medication by a doctor you'd met over text was far more palatable to many more people in 2022 than it had been in 2018. A Silicon Valley entrepreneur named Alicia Jackson raised $28 million from celebrities including Cameron Diaz, Gwyneth Paltrow, and Abby Wambach for Evernow, a women's telehealth company willing to diagnose menopausal symptoms and prescribe HRT by text. Fulenwider had launched Alloy by then, and Naomi Watts launched a skin-care and supplement company aimed at menopausal women featuring all sorts of moisture-replenishing products with punning names: Mask Me Anything, Vag of Honor.

The piece I wrote was titled 'Welcome to the Menopause Gold Rush,' and a few weeks after it was published, I got a call: Oprah had read it. She would be hosting a conference on menopause at the Hearst Tower in New York City, all to be streamed on her OWN network. Would I come as her guest?

Conference attendees were described as 'Oprah superfans of menopausal age from the tri-state area.' So many women patting their foreheads and patiently waiting for Oprah, Drew Barrymore, Maria Shriver, and Dr Sharon Malone, an ob-gyn who has discussed Michelle Obama's menopause on her own podcast, to take the stage. These women, and their specific moment in life, were being centered, and the thrill was palpable.

We all sat, nervously sipping on miniature bottles of Poland Spring. An executive from a big pharmaceutical company approached me. 'Thanks for the article,' she said. 'We're so excited about HRT.' She pumped her fist a bit.

In that context, my next question counted as small talk. 'So do you take it?' I asked.

'Oh, hell no!' she said, laughing. 'I tried for, like, two weeks and I just wept every day!'

She patted my arm and moved along.

Kooks

Oprah arrived, throwing her arms out and radiating charisma, warmth, and charm in waves so powerful they were almost visible. She told the story of her own menopause, which she says for years zapped her legendary mojo, left her feeling uninspired and blah. Gayle King, Oprah's best friend and *Oprah Daily*'s editor at large, chimed in with a funny story about getting her period all over a date's fancy car, and every woman in the room nodded in recognition: Who among us has never bled somewhere embarrassing and unintended?

When Oprah and Gayle started taking HRT, though, everything changed. Their moods! Their memory! Their minds all returned to their more essential versions: they became their younger, premenopausal selves once more. Life began to feel good again.

Their stories were echoed by Maria Shriver, by the superfans of menopausal age every time they got their hands on the mike. What I had previously understood as a complicated treatment that might offer some relief to some number of people for some period of time took on the air of a miracle. This was a fancy conference room on the roof of a Manhattan skyscraper, but it was also a revival tent: HRT was going to deliver us all. It was going to stop our hot flashes and fold our laundry and do our taxes. It was going to spoon us at night, reassure us that everything would be just fine, suspend us in the moment when our bodies were the best they'd ever been. It was going to suspend us there forever.

When the conference ended, I got five minutes alone with Oprah in a conference room. We held hands; we talked about Maya Angelou's menopause.

It was so overwhelming, it was all so *optimistic*, and it wasn't until I got about ten blocks from the Hearst building that I realized how strange it had all been, how little room this type of medical conversation leaves for the gray, for the complicated truth that many medical interventions help some people sometimes with some symptoms, but that this reality does not make for great television. Also, that aging is different from disease and that it isn't necessarily something to be *cured*. Again, not great television. We like stories, we like narrative, we like things to have beginnings, middles, and ends: a problem, a struggle, a resolution, an *arc*. Bodies and lives don't always comply, even when episodic television demands that they do, even when the market would like them to. The swell of the narrative arc is so alluring and so tempting, and there is no better narrator on earth than Oprah. How I longed for her version of menopause to be true for everyone! How I longed to live in a world not free from problems – ridiculous, that – but full of solutions! Neat, tidy, attainable solutions.

CHRONIC ILLNESS

One middle-aged rite of friendship passage is the sharing of ailments. It often happens over meals, but it can happen in other contexts, too. At work. Watching children do sports. And so on. It can concern gallbladders or skin. The refusal to drink, or the returning of a dish to a kitchen, or a sweater to a rack in a shop (wool allergies or sensitivities and so on). It can be an ailment that belongs to the woman herself or to her child. Floppy muscles or joints that bend too much or too little or systems that can't integrate certain enzymes or light. There are at this writing 5.3 million Instagram posts tagged #chronicillness. They feature candid photos of life in hospitals: tubes, bags, wires, and scars. Ostomy Awareness Day was marked, for example, with an image of a cute panda cartoon labeled 'Taking care of yourself is how you take your power back,' a sentiment that is repeated over and over and over again on posts about chronic fatigue syndrome, Ehlers-Danlos syndrome, lupus, irritable bowel syndrome, and chronic Lyme disease.

'I have never been well,' wrote the actress and writer Lena Dunham on the @sicksadgirlz Instagram account, captioning a series of photographs of herself tearful in a hospital gown. 'I don't know what people mean when they say "I'm fine." I am acutely aware we all suffer and I'm not some special pixie with pelvic issues, but I also know pain is isolating. And that isolation can be awful but it's also what makes me a writer and an artist and an empath. It's what makes me love to dance and paint and kiss and it leads to big triumphs and big mistakes and living big. I try and create awareness wherever I can for the issues I live with – OCD, endometriosis, Ehlers-Danlos syndrome, fibromyalgia, chronic Lyme. But I also worry it's too much of a mouthful, that nobody will believe so many diagnoses because ya can't get struck by lightning twice. It's all interconnected, I explain. I'm the scientist, the historian, the comedian – just trying to figure out how. Love, @lenadunham.'

The online culture of sharing has changed many aspects of what we know and understand about one another, and this is particularly true when it comes to the sharing of personal, formerly private struggles. Those who suffer from chronic illness are some of our most visible avatars of unwellness today, perhaps because, in the sharing of their stories and symptoms, many have found a vital combination of crowdsourced treatment knowledge and, at least as precious, the validation that they are not alone.

Historically, no one has been more ill-served by traditional Flexnerian medicine than the sufferers from chronic illness, who are, by no coincidence, usually women. The interrelated complexity of their conditions has gone undiagnosed, the reality of their pain has been ignored, the persistence of their symptoms has been dismissed. For these people, comparing holistic treatments, exploring functional medicine, sharing stories, and trading data are pursuits with the stakes of survival.

Many people with chronic illness call themselves 'spoonies,' a term coined by a Long Island woman named Christine Miserandino, whose ButYouDontLookSick.com blog was born of her frustrations in navigating the world with lupus. During lunch at a diner with a friend, Miserandino came up with the spoon theory to explain the limits on her energy that result from her chronic disease. She handed her friend a pile of spoons and asked her to think of each as a unit of energy. The number of spoons held by any individual on any given day represents the state of her disease: sometimes she might have a dozen, another day just three or four, and even the simplest acts – showering, driving to work, making the bed – claim some number of spoons. Miserandino wrote an essay about the conversation, and it caught on; google it and some of the first hits come from the Cleveland Clinic and WebMD. *The Daily Beast* described 'social media's latest conqueror' as 'the Chronic Illness influencer,' citing the increase in followers of Instagram and YouTube accounts held primarily by women who describe their often invisible diseases.

Spoonies find each other in online chats, and in person, too. There are spoonie meetup stations at conventions and concerts. According to the CDC, six in ten adults have a chronic disease, with four in ten having two or more, so it's not surprising that some spoonie Facebook groups have more than 100,000 members, or that spoonie videos on TikTok have garnered more than four billion views.

The illness memoir has grown off-line, too, as a literary genre. In *Sick*, a memoir by the writer Porochista Khakpour, the author is pictured on the cover with an oxygen cannula beneath her nose. She writes in the first chapter, 'The one thing I do know: I have been sick my whole life. I don't remember a time when I wasn't in some sort of physical pain or mental pain, but usually both.' The book is a winding and frustrating tour of Khakpour's difficulty getting a diagnosis for what is finally determined to be late-stage Lyme disease. Along the way, her relationships with family and friends and work are strained, and often entirely broken, and she is often not believed. She writes:

> It is no coincidence then that doctors and patients and the entire Lyme community report – anecdotally, of course, as

there is still a frustrating scarcity of good data on anything Lyme-related – that women suffer the most from Lyme. They tend to advance into chronic and late-stage forms of the illness most because often it's checked for last, as doctors often treat them as psychiatric cases first. The nebulous symptoms plus the fracturing of articulacy and cognitive fog can cause any Lyme patient to simply appear mentally ill and mentally ill only. This is why we hear that young women – again, anecdotally – are dying of Lyme the fastest. This is also why we hear that chronic illness is a women's burden. Women simply aren't allowed to be physically sick until they are mentally sick, too, and then it is by some miracle or accident that the two can be separated for proper diagnosis. In the end, every Lyme patient has some psychiatric diagnosis, too, if anything because of the hell it takes getting to a diagnosis.

There is also Meghan O'Rourke's *Invisible Kingdom: Reimagining Chronic Illness*, in which O'Rourke undergoes a similarly expensive and ultimately unsuccessful journey to figure out what is wrong with her, coming up mostly dry. 'One of the punitive fantasies – to borrow Susan Sontag's phrasing – society has long held about women who are ill is that their unwellness is mainly in their heads. The stereotype of the sickly woman whose disease is strictly psychological still holds today, when examples in medical literature of "problem patients" are nearly always women.' In Sarah Ramey's *Lady's Handbook for Her Mysterious Illness*, we meet Ramey, a funny, accomplished (she was a speechwriter for Obama) musician who struggled with chronic pain and unbelieving doctors for a decade. Ramey describes these mystery illnesses as 'the climate change of the human body.'

Maya Dusenbery wrote a well-researched book that includes the story of her own struggle with rheumatoid arthritis called

CHRONIC ILLNESS

Doing Harm: The Truth About How Bad Medicine and Lazy Science Leave Women Dismissed, Misdiagnosed, and Sick. It's a haunting journey into how unequal health care has typically been in America for women and especially women of color, and how powerful alternate online worlds have become for information sharing. Suffering the Silence, a non-profit founded by two women (one with Lyme, the other with lupus), is a platform for sharing stories of chronic illness that has even begun microfinancing for artists to tell their illness stories. A series of portraits feature attractive and diverse young people with their diseases written in bright white ink on their arms along with captions telling their stories. 'Every day I'm trying to learn to love a body I can't control,' reads one. 'The problem I had with my doctor was that I would go in complaining of pain and he said, everyone goes through this, it's called a period.'

A common refrain among the chronic illness influencers is that the search for alternative treatments is a necessity rather than a choice, the by-product of having been ignored and mistreated by the establishment for a terribly long time.

'Something I find frustrating,' Maya Dusenbery told me, 'is that there's not a recognition that people are not turning to these alternatives unless they are really desperate and have exhausted what mainstream medicine can offer. There are millions and millions of women who have conditions that are so poorly understood it's a misnomer to say that women are looking for *alternatives*.' Ramey has said that being described as a 'warrior' is unwelcome: How much better would it have been to just be treated? 'It's not that women come in and are always dismissed out of hand,' Ramey told *Salon*. 'It's that when the tests come back negative, then the default – in my experience and the hundreds of women that I've interviewed – is, "If we can't figure it out with the tests that we have available, then it must be psychological."'

Khakpour, O'Rourke, Ramey, Dusenbery, and the women like them are often dismissed by many in the great tradition of the Victorian hysteric, and they are exploited by others offering miracle cures. 'A jungle,' Ramey says, of people promising to heal and cure and explain.

The presence and the honesty of these women imply that their opposite must exist, too: Once we are no longer suffering in stoic silence, we become able to imagine the transcendent opposite. Once everything is out in the open, can't we fix it? Can't there be a solution?

And indeed, it does seem simultaneously possible and Sisyphean:as these conditions are treated, new ones are simultaneously named. It can seem both better and worse at exactly the same time, depending on the angle.

SELF-CARE

In 2021, *The New York Times* invited readers on a '7-Day Well Challenge.' Day 4 was devoted to self-care. 'What's the most important lesson of pandemic life?' Tara Parker-Pope asked. 'I would argue that it's this: Self-care isn't selfish... One of the challenges of 2021 will be to continue making self-care a priority once the pandemic has passed.' The first suggestion was to give the 'best hours' of the day to yourself. 'Giving yourself time every day to focus on your personal goals and values is the ultimate form of self-care.'

Before the late 1960s and early 1970s, 'self-care' was a term used mostly inside the medical profession to determine what level of independence was possible for vulnerable people (the elderly, the disabled, the mentally ill). Could they bathe themselves, prepare a meal, hold a job, hold a fork? It was a diagnostic tool with few implications for the mainstream population. Self-care, then, was literal health care; all the rest – manicures, massages, cleansing breaths of sea air – was grooming, or vacation, or something else entirely.

During this time 'self-care' also expanded to include people who work in high-risk and emotionally difficult professions, like EMTs, doctors and nurses, clergy. It was considered a necessary practice for caregivers to be able to do their jobs: a hospital chaplain who works largely in palliative care, for example, might require a constant monitoring of her emotional state in order to remain of service.

With the rise of the feminist and civil rights movements came the question of who was administering care and who was getting it. Women or minorities were not the answer to either question.

In 1971 a woman named Carol Downer was working with a Los Angeles chapter of the National Organization for Women, or NOW. She had six children of her own and had also endured a painful and illegal abortion while going through a divorce: a traumatic event that led to her becoming active in the pro-choice movement. Through NOW, Downer joined a group of women on a visit to a man named Harvey Karman in Los Angeles, where he was (illegally) providing abortions using a 'menstrual extraction' technique that was far safer for women than the scraping that was common in unprofessional procedures and that could result in infection and death.

During that visit, it occurred to Downer that after the six children and the abortion she had absolutely no idea what her own cervix looked like. Downer decided to 'borrow' a plastic speculum from Karman's clinic. She brought it home and, with the help of a mirror and a flashlight, took a good long look inside. How miraculous, she thought. And, why have I never looked at the entirety of my own body before? Downer was soon demonstrating how to have a look at one's own anatomy – often to dozens of women at a time packed into a small feminist bookstore – and considering which aspects of care and which procedures women might begin handling safely themselves. She and her group began performing exams on one another; they were not doctors, but they learned how to tell if something was not right. Most crucially, they were committed to treating each other with dignity and respect.

In 1970s in America, 93 percent of ob-gyns were men.

Self-Care

Downer and her partners believed that women knew intuitively how better to care for themselves and each other and that they were better equipped to take one another's concerns and complaints seriously. As they began helping one another with routine matters like yeast infections and more complicated ones, like the menstrual extraction technique for abortion, her theory was proven correct. They called this self-care, too.

Downer and a woman named Lorraine Rothman opened the first self-help clinic – the Feminist Women's Health Center – in Los Angeles and then took the clinic on the road, traveling across the country with a box of specula marked 'Toys,' teaching women how to examine themselves and about procedures like menstrual extractions.

In 1972, during a police raid of the health center, Downer was arrested in what was called 'the Great Yogurt Conspiracy' (they were using yogurt to treat yeast infections) for operating without a medical license. A jury chose to acquit, and soon after, when *Roe v. Wade* made abortion legal in America, Downer wasted no time: within sixty days the Feminist Women's Health Center clinic in L.A. reopened and was soon providing abortion services.

Some aspects of the self-care movement, like female reproductive health practitioners, have been absorbed into the mainstream: in 2018, 82 percent of ob-gyns placed in hospital residency programs were female.

Around the same time that Carol Downer and Lorraine Rothman were traveling the country in a Greyhound bus, the Black Panther Party (BPP), which sponsored a series of initiatives to fill the gaps left by the U.S. government when it came to caring for the poor and oppressed, was operating a series of 'survival programs'; the idea was that the failure to provide adequate nutrition and medical care to a significant portion of the population meant that that population was unequipped to fight back, to provide meaningful resistance against a system that was doing active and nefarious harm. A poster released by the Berkeley, California chapter of the Black Panthers read: 'A person's health is their most valuable possession. Improper health care and inadequate facilities can be used to perpetrate genocide on a people. The present fascist, racist government used its facilities for that purpose – the genocide of poor and oppressed people. The people must create institutions within our communities that are controlled and run by the people in order to insure our survival. With this in mind, the Black Panther Party announces the opening of our first Free Health Clinic in the Bay Area.' The text was accompanied by a drawing of a young Black child clutching a doll while an attentive Black doctor bandaged his arm. Central to both movements was the notion that women, particularly poor and nonwhite women, are frequently put in the caregiver position, with their own needs coming last.

The staff at the Panther clinics were volunteers, and they could be fired by their patients. The volunteer physicians were also required to undergo a form of reeducation. The BPP felt that any individual in a position to receive a medical degree could not understand the struggles of the people they were treating, so they provided a reading list that included works by Mao Zedong, Che Guevara, and Frantz Fanon.

When Arline Geronimus, who is now a public health professor at the University of Michigan, was a student at Princeton in the late 1970s, she had a part-time job at a school for pregnant teenagers in Trenton, New Jersey. The students were mostly minorities, and they were all poor. Geronimus began to notice the ways – big and small – that the students' health differed from that of her classmates at Princeton. Although the school treated their pregnancies as 'the problem,' Geronimus began to see it differently: the pregnancies, she realized, were often welcomed by the girls. The *problem* was the acute stress of living every single day with racism and poverty. Geronimus went on to study the long-term health effects of chronic poverty and racial discrimination on women in the United States and coined the term 'weathering,' which describes the cumulative effect of all this stress on the women (and men) who endure it.

What self-care was for, according to Geronimus and others, was preserving health and selfhood in a world designed to strip people like her teenage students of both. In a 1988 collection of essays that were written largely while she was fighting the cancer that would kill her, the poet and activist Audre Lorde wrote: 'I respect the time I spend each day treating my body, and I consider it part of my political work.' In the epilogue, Lorde writes,

> Sometimes I feel like I am living on a different star from the one I am used to calling home. It has not been a steady progression. I had to examine, in my dreams as well as in my immune-function tests, the devastating effects of overextension. Overextending myself is not stretching myself. I had to accept how difficult it is to monitor the difference. Necessary for me as cutting down on sugar. Crucial. Physically. Psychically. Caring for myself is not self-indulgence. It is self-preservation, and that is an act of political warfare.

Of course, it can seem funny that this once overtly political language is being used to sell massages and manicures, fluffy slippers and expensive sweats.

When 'self-care' began to enter the cultural lexicon, Americans outside the medical world were far more familiar with 'self-help,' with *Who Moved My Cheese?* and seminars where one can walk on hot coals toward a better, happier (and usually richer) life. Self-help implies the process of pulling oneself, hand over hand, to a higher position in the social or economic order, or even just to safety on a different shore.

Self-help has a long and robust American history, beginning with the publication of Samuel Smiles's *Self-Help* in 1859, which opens with the phrase 'Heaven helps those who help themselves,' which was really just a slight variation on 'God helps them that help themselves,' included by Benjamin Franklin in his *Poor Richard's Almanack* a hundred years before that. It was a maxim that would pave the way for success for people like Dale Carnegie, whose *How to Win Friends and Influence People* was first published in 1936, and Napoleon Hill, whose 1937 publication of *Think and Grow Rich* proved its own point by doing what it promised, for its author at least. The idea was that you could maximize your productive capacities: Speak louder, shake hands with more of a bone-crunching grip. Sleep less, do more. *Win.* Alcoholics Anonymous, which was founded in 1935, also started picking up steam around that time, largely because its method of treating alcoholism with a combination of spirituality, community, and talk was turning out to be more successful than any hard-medical intervention. It's the combining of these two disparate ideas that gives us wellness: that one could control one's health in an active, participatory way.

The new wellness definition of self-care is a hybridization of self-care and self-help more than it is exactly one or the other. What Geronimus began to notice, as self-care began to be co-opted by the wellness and beauty industries, was how recklessly the term seemed to be used.

'I think for the first time you have people who are very privileged for whom it is a very new thing to feel marginalized,' Geronimus says now, 'or who don't understand for the first time in their lives how the world could be going the way it is. Self-care was never about "avoiding triggers," or about "I deserve this." It was about finding protection from a world that was

Self-Care

really harming me. It's not *I've had a crazy stressful day so I should go get my massage,* or *I don't know how Trump got elected and I can't take it anymore, so maybe I should get a facial.*'

Audre Lorde's assertion that 'caring for myself is not self-indulgence. It is self-preservation, and that is an act of political warfare' is one of the most retweeted, Instagrammed, quoted, and misquoted texts in this entire community. The truth is, many instances of what is now considered self-care are not in fact acts of political resistance or rebellion at all.

Today, still, the biggest risk factor for poor health in America is belonging to a marginalized group. A 2015 report on healthcare equity from the Urban Institute and the Center on Society and Health at Virginia Commonwealth University noted, 'The greater one's income, the lower one's likelihood of disease and premature death.' A Kaiser Family Foundation study concluded that the death rate for Black Americans due to COVID was 1.6 times higher than the rate for white Americans. According to the CDC, in 2021, Black women are three times as likely as white women to die in childbirth. These disparities exist regardless of their socioeconomic status.

There is some vague pay-it-forward notion attached to a lot of so-called self-care. The maxim goes that self-care isn't selfish, but it can be. If Lorde's argument is that when an individual who has been systematically neglected by society at large rejects this paradigm and elects to care for herself, it can qualify as a radical and even subversive position, what is it when a wealthy white woman does so?

Ivanka Trump writes with regret about her failure in 'treating myself to a massage or mak[ing] much time for self-care' during her father's first presidential campaign in her book *Women Who Work*. As part of her publicity blitz, she tweeted, 'Self-care is not selfish.'

★

In spite of what the sandwich board outside my local nail salon reads ('take some time for self-care, you deserve it!'), many manicures and other rituals of grooming are not in fact particularly political acts, and indiscriminately claiming them as such is a bit of a stretch. Sure, everyone deserves to care for herself, but acts of hygiene and grooming needn't all be read as political acts, or the entire idea risks becoming a farce.

PART II
GLOW

WELLNESS IS EVERY BIT AS much about looking better as it is about feeling better. What used to be called beauty has been widely rebranded as wellness, or even health, which might suggest they are interchangeable categories, which they most definitely are not. But the borders between wellness and beauty are now almost entirely porous, creating a space where the pursuit of medical alternatives aligns with the search for an ideal face cream and a naturally ageless face to smear it on.

Old ideas about beauty summoned deception. The 'self-care' oases of previous generations were lavish, lush, overt in their assertion that pampering was luxury, and so the most common design reference seems to have been Marie Antoinette's Petit Trianon on the grounds of the Palace of Versailles. At the salon of Mr Kenneth, the hairdresser behind Jackie Kennedy's original bouffant (and Marilyn Monroe's platinum bob), clients sat on tufted velvet chairs ornamented with billowing taffeta skirts. The walls and ceiling of the salon were wallpapered, and each station featured a bamboo mirror and a small, silk-shaded lamp. Beauty, in those days, lay in artifice – bouffant hair, lacquered lips, the girdled hips and waist, the pointy bra. The condition of your pelvic wall, the consistency of your feces, were not matters to be casually discussed. The idea was always that *real* women – that is, beautiful and alluring women – should be repositories of secrets and deceptions, each with her own magic kit of smoke, mirrors, and personal, private *magique*.

How quaint that now seems in this moment of transparency! To be beautiful is now not to spend the longest time in Mr Kenneth's chair; it is to purify oneself from the inside out, to reek not of phthalates, but to radiate self-love and clean pores and the by-products of a heavily populated gut. This elusive state is most frequently and ambiguously described with one word: 'glow.'

Glow is radiance. Glow is health. Glow is a palatable aspiration in a climate of body positivity and next-wave feminism. Glow means radiance of skin but also of soul (that manifests itself in skin. And hair. And vibe.). The term is so prevalent that it sometimes feels as if a simple replace-all function has been applied to the entire beauty marketing machine: *Alexa, find 'skinny' and replace all with 'strong'; find 'beauty' and replace all with 'glow.'*

There is no shortage of advice out there on how to get a glow. It might be achievable with enough leave-in conditioner or a 'luminescent' shade of blush and has become a common word in the marketing of face creams and body oils. Topical options out there range from Glossier's Super Glow to Dr Barbara Sturm's Glow Drops, which retail for $160, or Guerlain's Abeille Royale Bee Glow, which is slightly less *chère*. There's Glamglow's Glowstarter and e.l.f.'s Halo Glow and Elemis's Superfood Glow Priming Moisturiser and KORA Organics' Turmeric Glow Moisturizer.

Even 'dry brushing,' which is exactly what it sounds like – the vigorous scrubbing of skin with a stiff, somewhat punishing brush – is said to give glow: fans say the practice increases the drainage of lymphatic fluids and flushes the glow-inhibiting toxins from your system, which is almost certainly overstating the case – lymphatic vessels are deep under the skin's surface, far deeper than brush strokes, however vigorous, could possibly reach – but it does swell the skin up and turn it red, which, in some lights, counts as glow.

Collagen, which is the protein-rich connective tissue between bones, factors enormously in discussions of glow. Collagen is what makes skin look plump and dewy; it lubricates our joints so that they swivel rather than creak. Collagen stores deplete naturally as we age, and so the race by marketers to boost them up – to replace glow's inner motor – is intense.

Glow can also be ingested, in the form of Goop's Everyday Glow multivitamin or HUM's Hyaluronic Glow gummies, or Love Wellness's Good to Glow supplements. A woman could move from Bridal Glow vitamins on to Goddess Glow Collagen Peptides to Womaness Fountain of Glow. There are even Wild One Glow supplements for her dog. The makeup artist and cosmetics guru Bobbi Brown walked away from her Estée Lauder-owned namesake company on its twenty-fifth anniversary, earned a degree in integrative nutrition, and started Evolution 18, a line of supplements and wellness products that encourage beauty 'from the inside out.' 'The better you feel,' Brown says, 'the better you look.'

If you *really* want to glow, make your diet all about it. On wellandgood.com a dermatologist named Dr Angela Lamb explained that your skin must have the correct balance of microflora, that is, the bacteria and yeast balance, in order to achieve glow. She recommends 'probiotics, fatty acids, niacin derivatives, oat derivatives, ceramides and squalene,' while another post quotes Janine Mahon, who has studied Chinese medicine and believes that glow is best achieved through a protein-heavy diet. 'Food therapy enables us to nourish the skin directly,' she says, 'and protein rich food will build the integrity of the skin and create a luminous glow.' Still another post offers ten recipes featuring sun-dried tomatoes that are 'packed with potassium' and all but guaranteed to make your skin *glow*.

By now we're almost back to medicine, and the modern equivalents of Mr Kenneth's clients would expect no less. High-end pampering now mixes the nurturing with the clinical: clinicians in white jackets walking across soft Moroccan rugs. At the Well, the wellness club that started in New York but now has locations in Connecticut, Florida, and Costa Rica, some rooms are dedicated to functional medicine consultations overseen by Frank Lipman, while others are strictly for massages and facials and sound baths. The room with the tented dome is for meditation. It's a full-service operation: bone broth and Ayurvedic tea are available on tap. A foot rub is one service, and an autoimmune diagnosis is another.

'I think that shopping at CAP is the ultimate act of self-care,' Kerrilynn Pamer, the CEO of CAP Beauty, said. 'Treating yourself with products that are loaded with life force and vibrancy is a direct statement that you care about yourself.'

If you aren't loving and nurturing yourself from every possible angle and in every possible way, how could you expect to look even halfway okay?

In the 1950s only about 7 percent of American women colored their hair. But then Clairol ran an ad for hair dye that read, 'How long has it been since your husband asked you out to dinner?' Today, the number of American women who color their hair is around 70 percent.

'Edna's case was really a pathetic one,' reads a 1923 ad for Listerine, which goes on to explain that halitosis was the reason that poor pathetic Edna had lots of experience as a bridesmaid but none as a bride. Almost-thirty-year-old Edna didn't even know! 'That's the insidious thing about halitosis,' the ad says. 'Even your closest friends won't tell you.' Listerine *will* tell you and then save you right away. Listerine's sales were around $100,000 in 1921 before the Edna campaign, and more than $4 million six years later.

How To Be Well

Women are so used to being described to ourselves as less-than (not thin enough, young enough, pretty enough) and then (*right away!*) offered solutions available to those willing to make the effort and absorb the cost. The 'Edna' ad can read as quaint, a relic from an era when it was acceptable for national advertising campaigns to describe marriage as a woman's main ambition. But this cycle of defining a problem and selling the fix is alive and well: the tagline for a 2014 social media campaign for Veet waxing strips, for example, was called 'Don't risk dude-ness.' In a fifteen-second online ad that ran in the spring of 2018, a pretty woman notices, while hailing a cab, that her armpit hair has grown in since her last shave. '*Shit,*' she groans as she is transformed into an overweight, slovenly man, now grotesque in her revealing green minidress, with hair not only in the unshaved regions but on 'her' chest and chin. The taxi peels away from the curb without her – who on earth would pick up a woman with hair under her arms? In another short spot, her boyfriend panics in bed when he realizes she has prickly hair on her legs; his eyes bulge as he clutches the bedsheets to his chest, as if under assault.

These ads were met by outrage on social media and quickly pulled out of circulation, but it remains true that as frequently as women are told that health concerns are psychosomatic, they are also told that bodies in their natural, untended state are worthy of disgust. If we fail to purchase and faithfully use expensive beauty products ('*I shaved yesterday!*' is the lament of the prickly girl in the Veet commercial) on a strictly regimented schedule, we are undesirable, grotesque.

Wellness has positioned itself as a reaction against all this shaming. Glow, and its implication of inner good health, sells an optimistic idea that a healthy body could potentially replace the so-called beautiful body as the most desired state, and that good mental health has a positive physical manifestation not unlike a facelift or an eyebrow wax.

Cure

If you call the desired effect glow, you can skip using the antifeminist term 'youth,' even if the implication is the same. Bodies can be described as universally beautiful, even when the obvious goal is to be thin; it's a cat-and-mouse blame game in which marketers avoid easily derogative terms without the more complicated burden of changing the stakes.

Because glow is also, of course, another product out there for sale.

BODY POSITIVE?

In 2004, Dove soap launched a multiyear marketing campaign called the Dove Campaign for Real Beauty, which, according to its parent company, Unilever, and its advertising partner Ogilvy & Mather, had one objective: 'To make women feel comfortable in the skin they are in, to create a world where beauty is a source of confidence and not anxiety.' It was a far cry from Edna's bad breath: billboards featured women of various body types and 'normal' faces (in place of model faces), which appeared at the same time as the publication of the 'Dove Report,' a corporate study with a mission Unilever described as creating 'a new definition of beauty [which] will free women from self-doubt and encourage them to embrace their real beauty.'

The campaign and the report were in many ways a success. Sales of Dove rose from $2.5 to $4 billion over the coming decade, suggesting that perhaps women were tired of being called disgusting. The reaction was a bit more mixed than all that money would suggest. The campaign was criticized as a cynical move on the part of Unilever, which also sold SlimFast diet bars, Fair & Lovely skin lightening creams (not exactly a formula for 'loving the skin you're in'), and Axe Body Spray for men, whose ads feature an altogether different type of 'real beauty.' Pascal Dangin, a well-known fashion industry retoucher of photographs, told *The New Yorker* that the pictures for the Dove campaign had been manipulated. 'Do you know how much retouching was on that?' he asked. 'But it was great to do, a challenge, to keep everyone's skin and faces showing the mileage but not looking unattractive.'

Whatever the hypocrisies involved, the Dove ads marked a cultural shift in the mainstream portrayal of bodies, as well as in the idea that bodies of different sizes can effectively drive sales. Cynical? Quite possibly. But also it's complicated.

In its purest form, the body positivity movement tries to reposition size from its dominant spot in the matrix of power and desirability, to propose the not-so-radical idea that a healthy body is a successful body, regardless of the shape it takes. But 'glow' has also proven to be an extremely lucrative marketing tool for any number of brands that target women in mainstream culture, one that contains within it the power to effectively sell products with a less easily definable and more inclusive goal.

Other massive multinational corporations followed Dove's feel-good lead. Weight Watchers, founded as a diet program in 1963 by a housewife named Jean Nidetch, had always done exactly what it said on the box: encouraging members to keep track of what they ate (via an elaborate points system), weigh in weekly, and report on progress to a similarly struggling group of peers. It trundled along for decades, selling branded food products and employing celebrity spokeswomen like Lynn Redgrave and Sarah Ferguson, then Duchess of York. But by the fall of 2015, the company was in a colossal rut: ten straight quarters of declining sales reflected a culture in which shaming women about their weight had gone out of style.

Oprah to the rescue! In 2015, Winfrey announced that she was investing $43 million for a 10 percent stake in the company, which soon kicked off a rebrand initiative called Beyond the Scale that it said was more holistic in approach while still promoting weight loss as a must and keeping points and weigh-ins as crucial parts of the program. It wasn't enough, and in 2018 Mindy Grossman, then the CEO of Weight Watchers, led the company to rebrand as the ambiguous entity WW, avoiding the word 'weight' entirely and hoping that the repetition of that suggestive letter would be enough to connect to the less shaming world not just of weight loss but of wellness itself. Indeed, the tagline was 'Wellness That Works.' (Some staffers, exhausted by asking what the new *W*s stand for, took to calling it 'wait, what?')

The new mission statement read: 'We inspire healthy habits for real life. For people, families, communities, the world – for everyone. The rebrand reflected WW's commitment to becoming the world's partner in wellness. While WW remains the global leader in weight loss, it now also welcomes anyone who wants to build healthy habits – whether that means eating better, moving more, developing a positive mindset, focusing on weight... or all of the above!'

In 2018, I got a magazine assignment to write about the Victoria's Secret Fashion Show, which had been riding a cultural high since it launched in 1995: an enormous spectacle featuring very famous models like Heidi Klum, Gisele Bündchen, and Gigi Hadid in teeny-tiny lingerie as Top 40 artists like Jay-Z, Kanye West, Taylor Swift, and Nicki Minaj belted alongside them. The whole thing was televised after the fact, and its ratings were high: in 2011 the telecast show reached its peak with more than ten million viewers. It was a master class in normative beauty. Every model was tall and long-legged, a body matching a specific set of proportions. Long thighs and midriffs, breasts that jiggle-jiggled but did *not* fold, small noses, long hair, straight teeth.

When I went to the 2018 show, I was allowed (following an NYPD background check) into the backstage area, which was done up like a giant vagina: pink satin and hot rollers. Roving (male) photographers were encouraging the models, who were all wearing bras, underpants, and short, monogrammed satin robes that only partially closed, to jump up and down on the sofas. I was led by publicists to the company's top executives, and I asked them how they were responding to evolving ideas about beauty, about the entire event as the #MeToo movement continued to gather steam. One after another they bristled at my questions. The next day, following a string of negative public reactions to the show, the company pulled out of any further interviews. Not long afterward the company fired the same executives I'd met and a year later announced that they'd no longer stage these bombastic odes to the (for most) unattainable ideal.

By then Les Wexner, its parent company's CEO, was under media scrutiny for his long-standing relationship with the convicted sex offender Jeffrey Epstein. This further tarnished Victoria's Secret's image. It was sold to a new owner and in 2021 reemerged with a new identity: VS&Co. Its new ads offered this message: 'We now know beauty was always yours to define. We see you. You're multi-dimensional. Ever-evolving. *Real.*' Quick shots of various women flashed on the screen: here is someone pregnant; here is a woman in a wheelchair, with soft rolls in her abdomen, laughing and wearing only a black bra and a small pair of black underpants. 'We promise to advocate for you,' VS&Co says. 'Now and Forever.' Craven? Absolutely. Better for the world? Yes, also that.

The most evident result of the rebranding VS effort has been a ninety-five-minute documentary-style video called *Victoria's Secret: The Tour '23*, which is available for streaming on Amazon Prime Video. The disjointed film features some familiar VS types – it's narrated by Gigi Hadid, while Naomi Campbell and Adriana Lima also turn up – but also twenty 'global creatives' of diverse size, race, and gender expression, hailing from diverse locations including Tokyo, Bogotá, and Lagos. The results were hardly earth-shattering, but VS faces a fair amount of competition in the woke-lingerie category, and it is hardly the only big fashion company to get on the size-inclusion bus. On the high end, so-called plus-size models have walked runways for brands like Fendi, Versace, Chloé, Michael Kors, and Chanel, and some of these models, like Paloma Elsesser and Ashley Graham, have appeared on magazine covers. Victoria's Secret has also faced more direct competition in the form of Aerie, a mid-market lingerie brand that launched in 2014 with a campaign called 'Real,' and ThirdLove, which in late 2018 took out a full-page ad in the Sunday *New York Times* that read: 'It's time to stop telling women what makes them sexy – and let us decide.'

A positive development in all this is that the truly modern young woman might not, for the first time in a while, list weight loss among her ideals. But the Zen of body positivity is tested whenever there are transformations to see. *Us Weekly*'s 'Celebrity Post-baby Bodies: Hottest Before and After Pics' serves us quotations similar to this one from the actress Jennifer Garner: 'I stayed in really good shape the whole time I was pregnant, and I was really careful with what I ate but for whatever reason my body just wanted to gain more weight this time, and luckily this time, for whatever reason, my body wanted to lose it!' As if the body and the 'I' were separate entities, blessedly and mysteriously united in the project of getting small.

In this cultural landscape of *all-bodies-are-beautiful-but-look-at-her-now!*, stories began appearing about a new class of diabetes drug that was being prescribed off-label for weight loss. It's how, people speculated, Kim Kardashian fit into Marilyn Monroe's dress that she wore at the Met Gala; it's why your favorite, relatable sitcom star was suddenly posing for people in a bikini with both ribs and cheekbones sharp enough to cut cheese.

The drugs – Ozempic and Wegovy were the first – were the synthesis of years of research by scientists including, crucially, an endocrinologist at the Bronx Veterans Affairs Medical Center named John Eng, who was delighted to find that the venom of the Gila monster – a big, fat, scary lizard indigenous to the American Southwest – contained a peptide that he named Exendin-4 that could control feelings of hunger and satiety by regulating insulin. Humans have a similar peptide, but the effect of the Gila version lasts far longer.

It took about twenty years of development, and the cooperation of scientists and researchers all over the world, but we all now know how the story goes: Novo Nordisk, a Danish pharmaceutical company, won the race, patenting the active ingredient called semaglutide in the drugs Ozempic and Wegovy, getting to market first, with many competitors and sketchy compounders following suit.

The way this new class of drugs – called semaglutides – regulates insulin has the potential to change everything about the way diabetes is treated. But it's the way this new class of drugs regulates appetite that has the potential to change everything about the way bodies are treated.

As the stories about off-label Ozempic use gained steam – all those is-she-or-is-she-not photographs of Real Housewives and actors, all those trend stories about expensive meals being thrown away barely touched in the expensive restaurants in Beverly Hills and on the Upper East Side – two different friends texted me on the very same day: 'So is this the end of wellness?' The implication was quickly very obvious: If we can all opt to be skinny with something as simple as a shot, do we need to keep pretending about all the rest of it? That these choices are made out of health, or altruism, or feminism? Out of anything other than submission to some patriarchal idea about what just looks better in our clothes and also out of them?

Oprah went on Ozempic and donated her shares in Weight Watchers to the National Museum of African American History and Culture, apologizing for the role she'd played in the endless torment of diet culture.

How To Be Well

Was this it? Was it done?

Aubrey Gordon – the *Maintenance Phase* podcaster – has described herself as weighing 330 pounds and speaks candidly about the many challenges of being fat in America: about the medical care she is denied, the assumptions that are made about her life and her choices. Her episode on Ozempic is, she says, the darkest one she's ever done. When everyone started calling Ozempic the end of the body positivity movement, Gordon joked with her cohost about the need for people to just 'ask a fat person.'

'The vast majority of fat people were under no illusions about broader social acceptance,' she said. 'At best, people said fewer unwanted things about our bodies. It never stopped. We were never lifted up. We were never centered. All we got out of it was one Lizzo.'

But immediately after the articles about Ozempic ending fat people were published came the stories about a whole new version of ugly: stories about old Ozempic faces and saggy Ozempic asses and droopy Ozempic tits. Sunken cheeks, hollow eyes, so-called ghost butts, haunting beaches all summer. Harvard Medical School describes the symptoms of 'Ozempic face' as 'sagging jowls' and a 'hollowed look to the face,' and suggests plastic surgery as a fix. Less authoritatively, the *New York Post* ran a pre-summer feature on the women who thought that Ozempic would have them ready for swimsuit season, only to be rethinking their shares in party houses in the Hamptons and on the Jersey Shore.

The sinking feeling was this: female bodies were still going to be scrutinized and ridiculed no matter what. The brief hope I'd had that body positivity had settled in for my daughters' generation was, I realized, an absolute myth: their favorite store, Brandy Melville, sold clothing in only one size, and that size was tiny. Girls who didn't fit simply had to look elsewhere; never mind the store's massive cultural dominance, they were just excluded. The world hadn't gotten better at all, and now the fix was leading to a new category of mockery, both for lacking the willpower to get there on one's own and for bearing the telltale sagging signs of such moral laxity. It was as if the lack of purity were evident in the sagging hollows of their cheeks. No, Ozempic was not the end of wellness culture, because the thinness that it offered – sallow, sickly – was a chemical thinness. It was not a wellness thin; it lacked glow. It lacked morality. It lacked deprivation and suffering and strength. But still, it was thin, and thin still ranked above fat. A March 2024 report by Vogue Business found that size inclusivity on runways in all four fashion cities had declined just as quickly as it had begun, and there had been an incremental decrease in sizing inclusivity by retailers as well.

SEX POSITIVE

With weight loss no longer the explicitly stated (just the strongly implied) goal, every inch of the body is now available for improvement. 'What the Eyes Can Tell Us About Chronic Stress,' reads a headline on Goop. A headline on Well+Good advises on how to know if you've had 'a flawless poop.' Who doesn't want a perfect poop! Can I buy a perfect poop? Would everything be better if I had perfect poop?

One of the more ascendant categories in the wellness industry, and certainly one that promises glow as a by-product, is 'sexual health,' sometimes called 'intimate wellness.' It's a prominent vertical for an increasing number of beauty and wellness retailers, which now commonly sell elegantly branded dildos, vibrators, and lubricants along with face scrubs and expensive shampoo. The makeup brand NARS has counted Orgasm as one of its best-selling blushes since its launch twenty-five years ago; now the preferred product is the orgasm itself.

'Masturbation is medicine,' declared an e-blast from Shen, the Brooklyn-based clean beauty company where I buy exfoliating cleanser and a hideously expensive German cream for my face. 'Self-pleasure has been proven to be an incredible resource for stress management with its ability to stimulate your "happiness hormones" that physiologically reduce stress, improve mood and relax the mind and body,' the Shen newsletter continues. 'It has also shown a very positive impact on focus, sleep and a strong immune system. In fact, masturbation has been recognized so cognitively and emotionally beneficial, that it has been integrated into many therapeutic practices globally.'

This is not the first time the medical benefits of the female orgasm have been described. It's a recurrence of the idea that female pleasure cannot just be an end unto itself; it must also make the woman's health, both physical and mental, *better.*

For centuries, discussions on women's health fixated on an idea about 'hysteria' – a broad and vaguely defined condition that was most consistently described as featuring intense emotional states, most certainly originating in the uterus. In the Ebers Papyrus of 1550 BC (among the oldest extant medical documents), the condition is treated by placing stinky herbs at one end – the mouth or the vagina, depending if the uterus is thought to have lowered or raised – and lovely ones at the other, to coax the uterus back, like a cat or, indeed, a mouse, to its correct position. Plato, Aristotle, and Hippocrates (who was the first to use the term 'hysteria') were all in agreement that the uterus that failed to join with the male was a sad uterus. Hippocrates felt that sex could even 'cleanse' the female body, ridding it of the foul and malodorous humors that were likely to travel around a woman's interiors and drive her nuts.

Much of the recent pop-cultural understanding of ideas about medicinal masturbation comes from *The Technology of Orgasm*, a 1998 book by the historian Rachel Maines, who settled on the topic when she came upon early-twentieth-century advertisements for vibrator-like devices while researching a project on needlework magazines and then posited that they were used in this specific way. It was not an illogical conclusion to reach: marriage and sex as cures for hysteria had been going on for hundreds of years – the successful resolution of 'hysterical paroxysm' was thought to return women to a state of usefulness – but it turns out the vibrators Maines was writing about were more of the Theragun than the rabbit variety, for tight shoulders and necks and such. If women used them for other purposes, that is one thing. There is no strong evidence that doctors did so on their female 'hysteric' patients.

Still, *In the Next Room, or, The Vibrator Play*, a 2010 finalist for the Pulitzer Prize, by Sarah Ruhl was inspired by Maines's book, as was *Hysteria*, a 2011 film directed by Tanya Wexler and starring Maggie Gyllenhaal and Hugh Dancy. Incidentally, the climax (ha) of *The Road to Wellville* is when the female patients are treated to orgasm by a newer, younger, handsomer doctor, and the embrace of the vibrator by wellness retailers certainly feels like a part of the reclamation of the (particularly female) body.

'I never claimed to have evidence that this was really the case,' Maines told *The Atlantic* in 2018. 'What I said was that this was an interesting hypothesis, and as [a recent paper] points out – correctly, I think – people fell all over it. It was ripe to be turned into mythology somehow. I didn't intend it that way, but boy, people sure took it, ran with it.'

The new masturbation ideology places the treatment not in the hands of a doctor, or even in the hands of a partner, but like so much of wellness in the hands of the woman herself. And it's designed and marketed like mad.

The Goop Double-Sided Wand Vibrator looks like an ice pop or a karaoke microphone, with its cheerful pink head. Kiki Koroshetz, the wellness director of content at Goop, explained it this way: 'We spent serious time on the aesthetic. The final design is sculptural and there's a fun pop of color. If you're inclined to leave your vibrator on your nightstand, it might even bring a little joy just to see it there.' The 2023 Goop Gift Guide offers a 'Made You Blush' kit for $180, in which the vibrator is bundled with a tinted balm in a shade called Venus and three shiny lip glosses. The kit is described as 'everything you need for the ultimate goop glow.'

Sex Positive

The Vesper vibrator by Crave is designed to multitask as a necklace in silver or gold: an elegant phallic pendant at the end of a long chain. ('This quiet, rechargeable clitoral vibrator doubles as a sleek necklace,' reads the description on the Nordstrom website.) Dame, an industry leader in the chic sex-toy category that makes snappy-looking sex toys that tend to cost around $100, has also launched three more affordable products to be sold at Target. It's also common now for ranges of beauty products to include a vaginal wash and a lube; the menopause beauty lines do, and the organic ones, too.

This transparency, this idea that everything is up for improvement, that everything could stand to work and look a bit better, can be exhausting. If you didn't feel bad enough about a drooping sex life, you can now worry that in addition to feelings of loneliness or whatever else, the deficit is affecting your looks, your life expectancy, your general health. If you don't have a glamorous vibrator on your nightstand, well, no wonder you look like that.

CLEAN BEAUTY

Oh my God, the packaging! The front lines of cosmetic glow, however they make you look, feel, and/or smell, are beautiful. My medicine cabinet is full of natural deodorants not because they work particularly well, or because I believe there is a link between aluminum in deodorant and Alzheimer's disease (research on Alzheimer's has not found any connection, but it's a rumor with decade-spanning legs), but because they are beautiful to behold. Wildist's Tangellow comes in a printed cardboard sleeve so attractive that I use it to store pencils on my desk. Corpus deodorant's sleek mint-green tube is printed with subtle golden letters that look copied from the imprint on a Phoebe Philo-era Céline purse, because the woman with that purse would not use a Secret aerosol deodorant; it would be tremendously off-brand. My nail polish is *vegan*; I wash my face with ground organic rice that I mix with water to form an exfoliating paste. To have *common* products – with their aggressive cartoon fonts and color palettes – would suggest a failure to consider oneself deserving not only of safety but also of luxury, a failure to execute proper 'self-care.'

Inside these lovely containers, the rule of thumb for glow-inducing beauty products is that they be 'natural' in terms of both effects and ingredients. Since all bodies are beautiful, they'll promise 'your lips but better,' your skin but 'radiant' (clearer and younger), your hair but 'sun-kissed.' Skin care is the new makeup, they might remind you. And since internal well-being is so explicitly linked to looking good, they'll agree that artificial elements are verboten. This growing sector is 'clean beauty,' a so-called alternative presided over by an often-self-taught band of beauty vigilantes.

Some of the biggest brands in the clean beauty category are, like many of the entrepreneurs in the wellness space at large, launched by women who began studying the idea out of fear that they themselves and their families were in danger. Onda is a clean beauty brands curator that began as an online store run by a former fashion editor named Larissa Thomson, expanding to a small storefront with investment by Naomi Watts. The idea for Beautycounter came to the marketing executive Gregg Renfrew after she watched Al Gore's documentary *An Inconvenient Truth*. 'I thought I was using natural oatmeal body wash,' Renfrew told *The New York Times* of her lightbulb moment, 'and in fact I was putting toxins on my babies. I was just outraged. And I became truly obsessed with this.'

Renfrew learned that the last time any significant legislation was passed regarding safety standards in common beauty products was in 1938, and so she started doing her own research. 'Most people still believe that the Food and Drug Administration is protecting them in terms of personal care products,' she said. Renfrew compiled a list of 'NEVER' ingredients that on last count was twenty-eight-hundred strong, created a line of shampoos, soaps, and cosmetics avoiding those ingredients, and attracted investment by Bono and a private equity firm. In addition to a direct-to-consumer website and a storefront in New York City, Beautycounter products have been sold old-school Mary Kay style, friend to friend.

What better method than a trusted peer letting you in on a terrible, upsetting secret and then immediately offering a safer choice?

After eight years in business, Beautycounter was acquired by the Carlyle Group at a valuation of $1 billion. 'If you think we're just selling lipstick,' goes their tagline, 'you're not paying attention.'

The official jury is still out as to whether these products are quantifiably beneficial to your health, but the concept of 'clean beauty' has exploded: one out of three beauty products for sale in America is labeled, in some way, 'clean.' In 2023 that meant it was part of an $8.1 billion industry. By 2028, the 'clean beauty' sector of the global market is expected to be nearly twice that.

Like Beautycounter, a lot of these companies are relying on a small piece of inconclusive evidence, often to the consternation of the chemists who are tasked with reformulating the products. As Amanda Lam, a cosmetic chemist who works for a chemical distributor, told *Allure* magazine, 'Our job is to create a sunscreen that will protect you from skin cancer, but today we are also trying to create a product for consumers who are scared of using sunscreen.' While research has definitively and unequivocally shown that overexposure to the sun's UV rays is the primary cause of skin cancer, the jury's still out on whether chemical sunscreen poses a similar risk. In the meantime, many cosmetic chemists find themselves tasked with removing and replacing so-called problematic ingredients from products, even when they consider the often untested alternative subpar, and this is often from products that have no official record of negative effects.

Because Americans have so readily accepted the notion of organic food as superior, applying the same standard to skin care makes sense. Skin care that is 'safe' enough to eat is the messaging of Juice Beauty, a California company that uses 'food grade' preservatives in its products. ('The same types... that are found in snack bars in your health food stores' is the claim, never mind that snack bars are considered a no-no by many.) Juice Beauty worked with Gwyneth Paltrow on her Goop-branded products, which she ate on late-night television with Jimmy Fallon. They dipped McDonald's fries into face cream. They really cracked themselves up. 'Better on your face, probably,' Fallon said, and Paltrow clapped her hands.

The verdict on clean beauty is officially literally still out. Sephora is facing a class-action lawsuit regarding its 'clean at Sephora' designation. But there is no question that it operates on an all-too-familiar plane where safety and health are sold as luxuries rather than rights, and where the what-if component has the potential to truly terrify. Poor Bad Breath Edna just didn't get married, but this time you'll get cancer.

Or worse.

Also, as the market for skin care pushes ever younger and younger, with tween girls now describing elaborate, multistep skin-care routines on social media and clogging the aisles at Sephora, their mothers are comforted somewhat by the notion that their young skin is at least touched only by 'clean brands,' much in the same way that Johnson & Johnson promised purity to earlier generations with 'pure' baby products designated 'gentle.'

DRESSING TO BE WELL

AMERICANS HAVE ALWAYS APPRECIATED CLOTHING that connects to leisure activity; Ralph Lauren built an empire around the idea of dressing for a sport you are unlikely ever to play. Clearly, he was onto something: activewear is a $68 billion industry that accounts for 22 percent of all apparel sales in the United States. Yoga pants – stretchy, black, forgiving, kind – have become daily wear for a generation of American women who wear them to exercise but also just to exist, manifesting, in a Veblen-like way, their connection to fitness and well-being.

On one level this is an outgrowth of the body positivity movement. Ideas on how women should look and present themselves have evolved alongside feminism, since the first-wave feminist pioneers of the mid-nineteenth century in America advocating for women's suffrage also launched Victorian dress reform to put an end to the then-popular practices of painful corseting and 'tight lacing.' (It was also sometimes known as the rational dress reform movement.) Women seeking the right to vote felt oppressed by the many discomforts of the corset and were afraid of their 'internal organs being displaced' by tight lacing, as one dress pamphlet put it. In 1851, an activist named Elizabeth Smith Miller from upstate New York began wearing a far more comfortable outfit: pantaloons with a knee-length skirt. Not only could she now breathe and move freely, but she could also speak loudly and publicly about her cause. Miller showed her outfit to her cousin the suffragist Elizabeth Cady Stanton, who loved it and showed it to *her* activist friend Amelia Bloomer, who was the editor of *The Lily*, the first newspaper in the United States edited by and for women. Bloomer, early influencer that she was, promoted the new garment in her paper, and it became known as the bloomer.

Around the year 2000, yoga pants became the new frontier in unrestricted comfort dressing. As with the creators of the bloomer, the man who popularized yoga pants always knew that this item of clothing was never just about yoga or just about pants. They were and are a statement about women, about culture.

Lululemon was founded in 1998 by Chip Wilson, a Canadian American Ayn Rand fanatic who had taken up yoga earlier that year because of back pain. (Lululemon's first shopping bags would be printed 'Who Is JOHN GALT?') By then, yoga was so much a part of mainstream culture that it was perfectly reasonable that a person like Wilson would take it up, but what he realized was that even the upscale women at the studios did not have a trendy, comfortable, and flattering outfit for their trendy pursuit. He set out to fill the niche with an imaginary perfect customer in mind: a thirty-two-year-old professional woman named Ocean who earns $100,000 a year, is 'engaged, has her own condo, is traveling, fashionable, has an hour and a half to work out a day.' (Later descriptions of the ideal male Lululemon customer revealed that Ocean is for sure outearned by her fiancé.) What Ocean would apparently wear were on some days premium leggings made from a yarn called SeaCell, which Lululemon's early marketing claimed to be a seaweed-derived substance that relieved stress through osmosis.

The pants took off. Was it because wearing them announced that the wearer has a 'practice'? Was it because the stretch material Wilson used had the effect of slimming and smoothing any bumps on hips and legs? Was it because once you slipped into the embrace of so much blended Lycra, regular pants, with buttons and zippers and flies, just felt so... *crap?*

Wilson had his own theories. 'Women's lives changed immediately [after the pill],' he wrote in a blog post on Lululemon's website:

> Men did not know how to relate to the new female. Thus came the era of divorces. With divorce and publicity around equality, women in the 1970s/80s found themselves operating as 'Power Women.' The media convinced women that they could win at home and be a man's equal in the business world... Breast cancer also came into prominence in the 1990s. I suggest this was due to the number of cigarette-smoking Power Women who were on the pill (initial concentrations of hormones in the pill were very high) and taking on the stress level previously left to men in the working world. Ultimately, Lululemon was formed because female education levels, breast cancer, yoga/athletics and the desire to dress feminine came together all at one time.

Obviously... no. Those parts about breast cancer and divorce and 'Power Women'? Oh my God.

I would alter his theory like this: Lululemon succeeded because women were fed up with being uncomfortable in clothes designed to force bodies this way and that, and because exercise and fitness became aspirational enough pursuits that women wanted to suggest a relationship to them even outside of the gym.

In any case, Wilson *was* right that everything and everyone would, eventually, make way for these pricey, stretchy pants. Cynics pointed out that you don't actually need anything to practice yoga, that it was a tradition touched and influenced by asceticism and these expensive pants were anathema to yogic dogma. But what does asceticism have to do with American yogic practice, anyway? The prevailing dogma is wellness, and wellness doesn't mind luxury.

Wilson incorporated wellness mindset into his brand's identity. In the beginning, all Lululemon employees who had worked there a year were offered the opportunity to take a free self-help course at the Landmark Forum, which was a corporatized version of the 1970s EST movement, 'specifically designed to bring about positive and permanent shifts in the quality of your life' in just three days.

In the first Lululemon store I became conscious of – SoHo, late 2000s – there was often a woman in the window doing yoga in shorts that revealed, as she moved from pose to pose, exactly where she shaved. Once I went in looking for new gym pants, and this yogi reached out and held my arm, cocked her head, and said, with deep eye contact, 'And how much support does your belly need? How much do you like to be held?' It was certainly a retail experience like none I'd ever had.

Douglas Atkin, the author of *The Culting of Brands*, once told *Fast Company* regarding Lululemon, 'It's the first time I've heard of anyone almost directly using the techniques of cults and applying them to their business.'

As with any cult, there were some credulity-stretching claims. The claim that the fabric used to make its pants came from seaweed and siphoned off stress was debunked when a hedge fund manager brought her pants to a lab for testing, figured out it was all a great big lie, and called Louise Story at *The New York Times*. The *Times* did its own investigation and 'found no evidence of seaweed in the Lululemon clothing.' The company's stock price wavered a bit, but then it rallied, and over the coming years another fabric – a trademarked matte nylon and Lycra blend called Luon – became one of its chief assets, its 'secret sauce.' In the end it was classic wellness branding: claim that the product makes you feel better, and if not, well, at least it makes you look better.

How To Be Well

Lululemon, which now has more than 650 stores around the world and a $6 billion valuation, has been knocked off at both high and low price levels. Customers who found the Lululemon prices too steep (pants tended to start at $98) found versions at Old Navy and the Gap. Designer customers were also pleased to see athleisure blending into their market: Stella McCartney, Missoni, Alexander Wang, Khaite, and Balenciaga have all collaborated with Adidas. Nike has made sneakers with the Japanese high-fashion brand Sacai and with Christian Dior and has even fashioned its iconic swoosh in Tiffany, robin's-egg blue for a limited edition Air Force 1 that sold out immediately, and now goes for four figures on the resale market.

Some designers were initially reticent about this development. I once interviewed Tom Ford in his aggressively *not* biophilic London atelier – Ford had always delighted in the hard artifice of glamour, and his office was all edges, lacquer, and frigid – and heard the resignation in his voice as he said that women 'need a beautiful coat and a bag because honestly, during the day, they're just wearing jeans. Or they're wearing their... *workout clothes.*' Pursuing wellness is such a big part of a well-off woman's life that it seems like folly for even the most exacting designers to exclude it.

The woman of athleisure now has many faces, many healthful pursuits beyond the yoga studio. Outdoor Voices, an Austin, Texas-based athletic wear company, targeted the millennial and college-age market who found Lululemon matronly, raising $57 million in venture capital funding around the notion of living well outside via the motto 'doing things *is* better than not doing things.' Outdoor Voices sent its products to ambassadors who posted endless images of themselves with the hashtag '#doingthings' like hiking up to waterfalls and doing backbends in their color-blocked Outdoor Voices gear.

Beyoncé's Ivy Park line of cropped T-shirts and bicycle shorts is for women who want to 'look and feel at the top of their game,' and when Rihanna first introduced her Fenty collection (which was later acquired as the first-ever female-founded fashion house in the French luxury conglomerate LVMH), she described the aesthetic as 'Marie Antoinette goes to the gym.'

Lululemon's most direct competitor, Alo Yoga, was founded by two men who practiced yoga themselves. It has grown to more than $1 billion in sales and come full circle to offering not only the clothes to wear for yoga class but also the yoga class itself.

Would Amelia Bloomer and her fellow corset rejecters be delighted to hear that athleisure is now what lots of American women wear almost exclusively? So much early fashion was predicated on the idea that the frailty of women meant they didn't need to move their bodies; to serve as an ornament was of much higher value. These are clothes *for* moving, and they are available in a range of sizes, with models to fit: Fabletics, Athleta, and Lululemon all feature models of various sizes on their online retail sites and mannequins of various sizes in their stores.

At the same time, one could argue that the athleisure ideal is its own kind of restrictive. If you're not coming to or from the gym, you should still probably be thinking about it. And society hasn't moved so far away from the idea that the ideal female body is a corseted one, even if that corset now comes in the form of calorie-restricted, strengthened abdominal muscles, as exhausting and often uncomfortable to maintain for many women as its tightly laced external predecessor. Women didn't really stop corseting; we just put the corset beneath our top layer of skin, to be shown off in spandex that, at whatever size, is always tight.

A corrective to this was pandemic fashion, which saw the extreme elevation of sweats — a piece of clothing Karl Lagerfeld once described as what a woman puts on when she has officially 'given up.' The new sweats outlived the lockdowns by growing only ever more luxurious: logo'ed Gucci tops and bottoms, shearling and mitten slipper-slides, fringed alpaca shawls, all a signal that this wearer is capable and deserving of self-care.

High-end shopping sites like Net-a-Porter and mytheresa.com have 'at home' and 'relaxed dressing' categories. A cashmere romper suggests a wearer in harmony with herself, putting her comfort and well-being before anything else. Loungewear carries with it the unspoken message that its wearer is, in all probability, very, very well. And thank God: please, someone, give that well woman a pair of elasticized pants, let her stay home, let her take a nap.

Just as her athleisure shows that she's glowing up in her off-hours, the well woman's travel plans are a time for serious renovation. The old umbrella-in-your-drink model that the travel industry used to refer to as 'fly and flop' is no longer as attractive to these women as are vacations as opportunities for self-improvement: a little light weight loss, a little acquired 'glow.' The Global Wellness Institute predicts a 16.6 percent growth rate for the wellness tourism industry over the next few years. Returning from vacation with a little pasta bloat is no longer acceptable: now one is expected to return rejuvenated, cleansed, purged, detoxified, and generally reborn.

For a long time, the most fashionable wellness retreats in America were the Ashram, in California, where attendees lived a famously spartan existence, sharing bare-bones rooms, taking long hikes in the baking sun, and existing on small numbers of carefully meted-out almonds, or We Care, a retrofitted motel in the desert outside L.A. where guests famously flopped around the pool, too depleted to do much more than describe the contents of that day's colonic. These places reeked of punishment and deprivation, of penance paid for crimes done in the course of regular Life. They were not vacation; they were corrective.

Dressing to Be Well

This has all changed.

Big chain resorts and small boutique hotels alike list their 'wellness' offerings alongside their accommodations and rates, and these offerings extend beyond spas or gyms with a stationary bike and a sad stack of free weights. Westin Hotels has an elaborate wellness plan that 'empowers guests to transcend the rigors of travel while on the road through the brand's Six Pillars of well-being: Sleep Well, Eat Well, Move Well, Feel Well, Work Well, and Play Well.'

Yoga mats are widely available, and so are maps featuring highlighted jogging routes. More and more hotels have pillow menus to accommodate all types of sleepers, and staff nutritionists to add 'superfoods' to room service menus.

And old-school European medi-spas à la *The Magic Mountain* ('our air up here is good for the disease — I mean good *against* the disease') have been experiencing a boom, fueled by influencers posting and tagging endless photos of themselves in big robes receiving IV therapies, dunking in brisk alpine lakes, and eating minuscule portions of beautifully sliced and diced raw food.

This can happen at the Lanserhof medical spas in Germany, where the mission is 'the thorough regeneration of the intestines to revitalise the vital forces,' plus lots of rest on high-thread-count sheets. Or the Mayr method, which is practiced at competing spas in Austria. The Mayr method, which has been around since the 1920s, involves eating very little food and chewing it for a very long time, and also getting rough stomach massages and regular colonics and, if Instagram is to be believed, regularly dipping in a nearby lake while wearing a $400 Eres one-piece bathing suit. The Viva Mayr clinic is known for its celebrities — Kate Moss, Elizabeth Hurley, Karlie Kloss, the Rolling Stones, even Theresa May! Rebel Wilson and Melanie Griffith and Jenna Lyons and Naomi Campbell and half of Bollywood have all partaken of the Mayr interval hypoxic hyperoxic treatment therapy, the saline inhalation, the vigorous this and the vigorous that.

The Chenot Palace in Weggis, Switzerland, is the latest offering based on the 'successful aging' teachings of Henri Chenot. Its old-school chalet-style hotel got an expensive renovation and a brand-new spa in 2020, setting it up as a perfect post-pandemic detox center.

For those who prefer a more hippie version – fewer hard-bristled brushes and freezing-cold showers – there are similar destinations in Ibiza, where the Six Senses resort features yogic masters and 'immersive retreats,' as well as hyperbaric oxygen chambers, cryotherapy, and tests to analyze your DNA, and where you might get to meet Mark Hyman. Joali Being in the Maldives, where villas go for upward of $4,000 a night, offers integrative health assessments ranging from the Ayurvedic to the high-tech.

And on, and on, and on.

GLOW LIFESTYLE

It's impossible to talk about any one piece of the wellness aesthetic — yoga pants, clean makeup, body positivity, Goop vibrators — without seeing how interrelated they all are. Each access point is an invitation to a lifestyle. The Glow Cinematic Universe, maybe.

There is a certain set of clothing labels designed by mid-career women who have bypassed the traditional fashion routes to sell directly to their customers online. The clothing sold by these brands is expensive, but it is far below the designer level, and it is still largely worn by white women on the coasts. The boast is of fair labor practices, progressive business models, and clothing built to last, as opposed to the trend of 'fast' fashion, which has proved to be an environmental catastrophe. Models are used to display clothing in catalog settings, but the interesting marketing side of the operations are shoppable 'diary' or 'journal' verticals that appear alongside the e-commerce. The women featured tend to be not models but 'real' women, well women, whose lives are versions (often aspirational versions) of the lives led by the potential customers. They are gallery owners, furniture designers, and photographers who live in glass boxes in the leafy canyons of Los Angeles, or in Brooklyn brownstones with thick-chipping paint and antique marble fireplaces. Always, their lives are described in relationship to how well they are: they talk about beginning their mornings with meditation, green juice, sun salutations. Many describe the importance of forgiveness, primarily the process of learning to forgive themselves for perceived failures and flaws.

The blog-journal at Shopdoen.com, which is the website for Dôen, a California-based 'collective' that sells prairie dresses and peasant blouses, showcased a former doula who now lives on a small island in Puget Sound, and another who devotes her life to the end of single-use plastics, and also Alyssa Miller, who lives in Hollywood on a 'city farm' with '3 dogs, 2 cats, 1 pig and 7 chickens.' Another entry features Kyle and Sian, of Love Yoga in Los Angeles, who suggest 'meditative breathing and touching every part of the body as a form of maintenance.' They wear Dôen while demonstrating headstands beneath the Venice Beach pier. On the Jenni Kayne blog, you can find articles on the benefits of spirulina, how to make a moringa power breakfast bowl or an invigorating coffee shower scrub, alongside the cashmere fisherman sweaters and pony hair slides on offer. A typical interview (this one with a physical therapist) reads: 'I wake up at 5:30 am so I can have a few minutes to myself before anyone else is up in my family. I often sit and do some breathwork, set my intentions for the day, and brew a pot of coffee. This routine helps me feel grounded and prepared for the day ahead.'

We have quickly expanded from upscale casual to an entire way of being.

'If imploding a successful life can be considered a radical form of self-care, consider Lavanya Mahendran's year,' read a post on the online journal of Apiece Apart, a small and cultish fashion brand favored by women who burn palo santo and make time to meditate. Mahendran, who was modeling a printed wrap dress, had been a senior-level executive at Google and a litigator until she decided to 'give in to the feeling of being uncertain' and take a yearlong journey around the world. The photos on the blog were taken during a stop in Mexico City. Another featured woman, Su Wu, who was photographed modeling a pale pink jumpsuit in the old theater she is renovating also in Mexico City, described the experience of her childhood best friend coming to Mexico to serve as her doula. 'She smoothed my edges, with flower petal baths, with cupping and acupuncture, and with soup made with seaweed she'd collected herself on the California coast. Then, after the birth, she took my placenta away with her in a mini cooler and entered a monastery.'

Apiece Apart ran a long feature on Sharon Mrozinski, a woman in her late seventies who divides her time between an island off the coast of Maine and a small market town in the South of France. Mrozinski is tall and athletic, with short white hair and a tanned, lined face. While she models a pair of high-waisted white cotton pants, she describes her work as the proprietor of both a small inn and an antiques shop and her marriage of some thirty-five years. 'We get up early and typically do yoga and meditate,' she says, 'and go for a walk and end our day the same way. We cook simple meals at home. We eat simply and live simply and work almost isn't work for me.'

Frequently, these subjects share intimate stories, about grief, for example, or addiction, and they also share the details of how they wash their faces, read to their children, and care for their guts. 'If there is one thing I've learned during my cosmic voyage to the depths of hell,' writes Molly Rosen Guy on the Dôen website of the year in which she got divorced and her father died, 'it's that you've got to treat your grief like a tender little preteen in a training bra. Speak to it calmly, don't make it go to loud parties, and let it spend lots of time doing quiet, cozy things around people who make it feel safe.' In the accompanying photographs, she modeled a long, dark $212 dress in a 'Black Prairie Paisley' print.

A few years ago Apiece Apart published a conversation between a creative director and a photographer modeling printed dresses atop volcanic rock on the Hawaiian seashore. It was centered around the idea of 'setting intentions'. 'Yesterday I did a loving kindness meditation,' says one to the other. 'Have you ever tried that? Such a nice practice of self-acceptance and compassion.'

These conversations would have been unlikely to have occurred in Mr Kenneth's limestone salon on East Fifty-Fourth Street, where the air smelled of polymers, nicotine, ethynol, and Chanel No. 5.

To be well, though, is not to be a prig, and ultimate wellness preserves a space for indulgence. There's plenty of talk about the beloved glass of (organic, low-tannin) wine, the long late night with friends that trumps the perfect ritual of sleep. 'We've gotten very focused on perfection masquerading as wellness,' the stylist Kristen Naiman told Apiece Apart. 'It's just another way to beat ourselves up.'

Told correctly, even smoking can be read as wellness. 'One cigarette a day is my guilty pleasure,' says Naiman. 'I don't do it every day and I go in and out of it for months at a time but I give myself an allowance that if I want I am allowed up to one cigarette a day. For me, why even have a guilty pleasure that's, like, four squares of dark chocolate. That's not a guilty pleasure! That's just necessary. A guilty pleasure should be something that's a little bad for you.' Meditation is all well and good, but 'allowing yourself to have some messiness, some living for now, not for later, is important.'

As Jenni Kayne evolved her business from pure fashion to wellness lifestyle, she found a mentor in Martha Stewart. At a dinner launching her book *Pacific Natural*, Kayne's guide to 'simple seasonal entertaining' that suggests crafting afternoons with friends to make jars of lavender honey sealed with pretty burlap tops, vegan blueberry muffins for picnics at Lake Tahoe, and homemade granola for mornings on the ranch in Santa Ynez, Stewart toasted Kayne. A disciple! The line was so clear from

Glow Lifestyle

Martha Stewart's tasteful version of entertaining – eggs from her own Westport chickens, baby gem lettuces grown in the fog on Mount Desert – it was possible to see exactly how it had influenced this generation. The notion of Martha Stewart was always that she did things *better* than everyone else, and that if only you had the time or the good taste, you, too, would churn your own butter on a charming antique bike. It was only laziness or other, generally 'bad' character traits that kept us from our 'good things' lives.

At the dinner party, I sat opposite Claire Olshan, who had founded a small, expensive, and beautiful boutique in a town house on Manhattan's Upper East Side but had moved on to trying out a collection of healthy vegan snacks she'd christened Dada Daily. She was especially proud of the crispy almond-butter Brussels sprouts and of the packaging, which was big and loud and designed to show up well on Instagram. 'It's really what I've always been passionate about,' she told me. 'It's probably because I totally had an eating disorder in high school!' (Six months after the launch of Dada Daily, Olshan gleefully thumbed her nose at the wellness aesthetic in favor of a surrealist, 'let them eat gluten-and-dairy-free cake' vibe. She threw a party in a Manhattan apartment that was listed at the time for $125 million, and guests were served Dover sole out of bedazzled $495 Jimmy Choo pumps.)

Everyone's skin was glowing. I recommended a chiropractor to someone with a stiff back. I overheard a debate on the efficacy of vitamin D drops versus vitamin D capsules versus going out in the sun, but no one looked as if they'd been in the sun at all; everyone's skin was so clean and fresh. Everyone looked as if the sage-scented candle from the goody bag had been lit inside their neutral cashmere sweaters; everyone had *glow*.

The Italian actress Isabella Rossellini lost her contract with Lancôme when she was forty-three years old. 'They told me they needed somebody younger,' she explained. 'The advertising was aspirational, and even though they have clients of many ages, the desire was for youth.'

So Rossellini took in a lot of foster dogs and studied for a master's degree in animal behavior and conservation at Hunter College and made a series of weird and hilarious short films about the different ways that insects have sex. Here was an interesting and engaged woman, pursuing her passions and living a rich and varied life, full of hyperlocal produce and the cultivation of bees. Lancôme, with a new female CEO, tracked her down on the South Shore of Long Island, where she runs a twenty-eight-acre organic farm specializing in chickens that lay eggs with exceptionally creamy yolks. Rossellini has not had plastic surgery. She works in boxy, rumpled linen clothing, has dirt beneath her nails. After a twenty-year hiatus, Lancôme realized what it was missing and signed her again.

There's something undeniably nice about virtually meeting these women, about seeing clothes modeled on their different sizes and shapes at all levels of fashion and retail. These images and ideas are far more like the aspirations that women actually hold for themselves. It is all a much more comfortable place to exist. The wellness aesthetic has appeared at a moment when artificial beauty is ascendant: social media filters, plastic surgery, *contouring*. The massively popular and influential Kardashian beauty ideal has little to do with health: the sisters got in trouble for endorsing QuickTrim, a weight-loss-oriented amphetamine-speed combination product that for a while was packaged with a picture of Khloé and Kim Kardashian and the tagline 'How hot can YOU be?' Khloé Kardashian has promoted meal replacement shakes called Flat Tummy by posting mirror selfies with her shirt off. They are often busted on social media for sloppy retouching jobs, forgetting to replace crucial body parts, like hands, arms, toes. They have lips that look too heavy for eating or talking; their positions in photographs look so uncomfortable to hold.

But these women on the volcanic rocks, in their prairie dresses and espadrilles, piloting wooden boats around Puget Sound and raising chickens within view of the Hollywood Sign, aren't kidding when they say they want to meditate, eat whole foods, walk naked in the woods. They are fed up and burned out, and in a privileged enough position to do something about it, to write a new story for themselves about how successful, privileged women should look and be and feel about themselves and their wrinkles and freckles and thighs.

And once again, here we are, reaching for something of which it is so easy to fall short. Here we are, again, attempting to spend our way to better selves.

PART III
SPIRIT AND SOUL

I AM A SECULAR ATHEIST most at home in the big coastal city where I live and other big cities like it. Despite my Jewish and Roman Catholic parentage, I have been to synagogue only for other people's bar mitzvahs, funerals, and brises, and to church only for weddings, more funerals, and the occasional boozy midnight Mass.

But for a secular atheist, with predominantly secular, atheistic friends, I am often on the receiving end of vague, quasi-religious pep and/or dharma talks from an ever-expanding group of unusually attractive strangers. In some instances, they know me only by the cryptic set of initials that comprise my username on the alarmingly public 'leaderboard' that appears on the right side of the screen during an at-home ride on my Peloton bike, where my fellow seekers have included Joe Biden, Michelle Obama, and David Schwimmer, whose name once flashed on my screen and then just as quickly disappeared as he left me in the virtual dust. Sometimes it happens in person, though the exchange is thoroughly one-sided and I am usually shrouded in the dark. If I am known at all, it is because I am consistent, a seeker of habit, registering always for the same bike in the same SoulCycle class, occupying the same inconspicuous back corner of the dance studio, often wearing the ignore-me uniform of matching black leggings and top.

If I consider the seminal events of my adulthood, these

demi-strangers have been a consistent presence: they talked me through the Trump years, COVID, the social unrest that followed the murder of George Floyd, the atrocities of war in Eastern Europe and the Middle East, the baffling mornings after of mass shootings, the rage I have felt at American political chaos. They have called on me to pray (I have never *consciously* prayed) for my fellow fitness freaks in their times of need, helping them 'manifest' new jobs or new relationships or new ways of looking at the world, and they have called on me (on all of us) to ride in solidarity with fellow stranger-classmates who are facing unspeakable difficulties: illness, loss, grief. They have asked that I join in breathless and ecstatic movement frenzies: shaking, shouting, screaming, and singing and dancing as a member of a vibrating mass.

In my grandparents' generation, the number of Americans who identified as Christian was 95 percent. Ninety-five percent of Americans were affiliated with some organization that would invite them to potluck suppers and sing-alongs, provide an opportunity to dress up and get out on the weekend, to see neighbors, to gossip, to worry, to funnel efforts into caring for one another and choosing to believe collectively in a set of explanations for the unexplainable parts of life. My maternal grandmother was both a proud Jew and a proud atheist to the very end, affiliated with the same synagogue as the group of women she met as a toddler and knew until she died at ninety-eight.

Times have changed. The number of adult Americans who identify as members of any organized religion has been consistently declining. That describes 95 percent of the members of the so-called greatest generation (born between 1901 and 1927) and the silent generation (born between 1928 and 1945), in contrast with 70 percent of the members of my generation – Gen X – and just 57 percent of older millennials (born between 1981 and 1989) who identify as Christians.

This is not because we suddenly have all the answers, or that the human inclination toward seeking has stopped or even slowed. As participation in traditional organized religion declines, the number of Americans who identify as 'spiritual' continues to rise. According to Pew Research, about 70 percent of Americans describe themselves as 'spiritual,' though 27 percent identify more specifically as 'spiritual but not religious.' SBNR is even a descriptive option on some dating apps.

Into this space has stepped the gospel of wellness. I don't know many people with organized religious lives, but I know many with strong rituals, routines, and communities that center on fitness. I know many people who have used exercise – and the community that comes with it – to get through a difficult divorce, the grief of losing a parent, the isolation of a lonely quarantine, who have accepted advice and counsel from fitness instructors (both in person and virtually) on matters of morality, community, and service. I also know people who consider Brené Brown's books scripture; who take cleanses as seriously as any purification ritual; who consult a range of astrologers and psychics and vaguely defined 'healers.'

Wellness is a ready home for many of today's SBNR. Its temples are places to make the body more whole, alongside the rest of your congregation. Its prophets are gurus preaching self-care and mindfulness. Its relics are crystals and horoscopes, totems with which to hope for a more attentive cosmos. If all this sounds a little scattershot, that's kind of the point; wellness spirituality is at once unified in its messaging (it's all about you, and you've got this!) and fully à la carte in its devotional options. *Namaste all day.*

SOUL

In 2015, two graduate students – Angie Thurston and Casper ter Kuile – at the Harvard Divinity School realized they were both interested in how millennials were redefining the spaces in their lives that would have been filled, in earlier generations, by church. As they wrote in a summary of 'How We Gather,' a study they coauthored, 'Millennials are flocking to a host of new organizations that deepen community in ways that are powerful, surprising, and perhaps even religious.' Together they looked at ten secular organizations that were, in some ways, mimicking religious institutions. They defined these organizations as epitomizing a combination of six themes: community, personal transformation, social transformation, purpose finding, creativity, and accountability. Among these organizations was SoulCycle.

When the stationary cycling fitness company SoulCycle was founded in 2006, the founders were aware that the yellow wheel they adopted as their logo bore some resemblance to the Buddhist wheel of dharma, but they didn't push that idea too hard. Including 'soul' in the name was probably enough to broadcast their intentions. SoulCycle's founders recognized the spiritual longings of upscale urban women and merged them with a new demi-yogic language in a setting committed to cardiovascular health. The founders were always aware of what it would mean to put instructors high up on an altar, lit only by flickering candles, surrounded by row after row of devotees.

From the beginning, instructors were told to indulge in as much feel-good talk as felt right. One of SoulCycle's first hires was Janet Fitzgerald, who described her job to me like this: 'I ask for guidance to put the music together in such a way that will help people feel strong, enthusiastic, good in their bodies, creative, uplifted, and I ask for words to move me through that will help transform and motivate. My soul calls for that. It's a calling.' Fitzgerald taught a Sunday morning class called Sunday Service, with adherents considering it an important weekly milestone for reflection and identity. The collective power of prayer is often invoked: Fitzgerald might ask the entire class to manifest the dreams of another rider, or send health to the sick, shouting, *'AND SO IT IS!'* once she detects the eyes closed and the energy focused strongly enough. One of her more common admonitions is *'RIDE AND PRAY! RIDE AND PRAY! RIDE AND PRAY!'*

Does this borrow from karma yoga – the notion that one's daily actions should mainly be of service to others? As fitness is uncoupled from the larger practice, it can work as a handy overcoat for narcissism: it can be embarrassing to spend so much time and money on oneself in such hideously unequal times, and this idea can offer a crutch for the conscience, or at least an attempt to recast these repetitive and narcissistic actions into honorable and tradition-bound performances of virtue and concern for one's fellow man.

'When I was freebasing cocaine and dating Israeli mafia, I probably didn't know much about the mind–body connection,' Fitzgerald once told me. 'But I have walked on fire, done breathing exercises, sat in sweat lodges, seen every healer known to man, drank ayahuasca in the deep jungles of Peru, and I have found nothing as transformative as that bike and what we do in here. So I always knew that if I could beat the shit out of people and then evoke emotion in the moment with certain kinds of music once they had been broken down a little bit that I could get people to open up, to cry, to remember who they are, to remember their story, their purpose on the planet above and beyond making money and losing weight.' (Not, to be clear, that I've found many people in spin class who aren't interested in the latter, and sometimes the former. The Peloton instructor Robin Arzon often starts her class with the warning that you might be so inspired at the end that you might 'hire a publicist! or register an LLC!' And I often think, *That would be nice, but losing five pounds would be enough. Really.*)

'We are *not* using my workouts as a distraction from reality,' the Peloton instructor Jess Sims (who looks so much like an anime character that my daughter once wondered if I was in fact taking class from a cartoon) says. 'We are using my workouts as practice. Physical practice to show ourselves we are capable of doing hard things. We are capable of getting uncomfortable and really effecting great change – within our bodies, within our minds, within our families, within our communities, and within our world!'

To become an instructor at SoulCycle, it is imperative that one graduates from 'Soul Day,' a candlelit meeting where trainees share stories of their struggles and traumas with the group – childhood abuse and neglect, poverty, addiction, cutting, in addition to the more abstracted forms of self-loathing and doubt – before taking their places on the altar.

How riding a bike to nowhere came to be attached to such profound personal and spiritual longing is not necessarily clear. The idea for indoor cycling as a group fitness exercise began in Southern California in the late 1980s after a competitive long-distance road racer named Jonathan Goldberg – Johnny G – who was recovering from an accident wanted to find a way to train in his own garage. Within a few years, Goldberg and his fellow cyclist friend John Baudhuin had designed a bike that was better suited to highly energetic, calorie-burning stationary exercise, and they began to teach classes, experimenting with the motivational effects of incredibly loud, 170-beats-per-minute music. They named this new exercise Spinning and founded a company called Madd Dog Athletics that both sold these bikes and offered classes led by the hopefully charismatic instructors they had trained. An audience developed fast: Spinning is a nice option for people who want to get all sweaty and out of breath without having to jump around.

I'd tried Spinning years before SoulCycle at a gym in my neighborhood – the instructor liked Madonna's *Ray of Light* album, and all anyone was doing in there was trying to look better nude. Why else would you go to the gym in a city where there was so much else to do? There wasn't some idea of a shared mission or purpose or philosophy or anything much except higher, tighter butts. The gym was like the dentist: unpleasant, but also necessary for maintaining a level of urbane personal hygiene. Eventually, I stopped going. I was too distracted by everything else available in the city when you are young and single with plenty of curiosity and time, but after my first maternity leave I was back at work feeling tired, sluggish, and slow. I went to lunch with a woman who was interrupted the whole time by texts from her SoulCycle teacher: 'u r beauty'; 'u r strong and brave and courageous.' There were also lots of emojis: hands clasped in prayer, hearts, halos, rainbows, stars. There was something intriguing to my exhausted, new-mother mind about the idea of bathing in so much easy positivity and affirmation and love and, frankly, selfishness. This wasn't language that was common in my New York life, and it certainly didn't resemble the drudgery and mild humiliation of the gym as I had previously known it. This woman signed me up on the spot for a class that weekend. 'It will change your life!' she said, with a pupil-dilating stare that both rattled and intrigued.

SOUL

I started with a class on a hot, sticky day while I was trying to wean. Sweat and breast milk were soaking my T-shirt; my stomach was soft and hanging over the band of my pants. 'I just had a baby,' I told the instructor apologetically. I pinched my stomach, offering up the type of evidence that had so excited the gym buffs in my past – *Ew! Gross! A project!* – but the instructor looked horrified. (The instructor was Stacey Griffith, who like Fitzgerald was once a drug addict, alcoholic, and admitted 'liar.' In her 2017 book she describes her SoulCycle classes as an opportunity for 'overcoming the issues in our tissues – the deepseated memories and learned behavior we get hung up on.') 'That is *beautiful*,' she said to me that day. '*You made a life.*' I was chastened. I was immediately buried in the very specific language of the place: moving back and forth over the seat to 'tap it back,' adjusting the resistance knob to make 'hills' in the dark as candles flickered against the walls. 'Addicted,' read one wall. 'Obsessed.' Elsewhere: 'Inhale intention. Exhale expectation.' News reports that Amy Winehouse had killed herself had come out a few hours earlier, so Griffith suggested we just 'ride it out for Amy' and be thankful for the air in our lungs and the beats of our hearts, and she wanted us all to know that she was there for us, any of us, if we ever felt down.

The current exercise guru barely mentions the body at all, except through the generous use of the increasingly loaded word 'strong', and endless iterations of the so-called airplane oxygen mask theory, in which one's own needs reign supreme and everyone and everything else – your family, income inequality, climate change – stand to benefit via some trickle-down effect. *How are you going to carry this energy and this feeling forward?* Spin instructors often ask at the end of class. *How are you going to spread this energy around?* 'You're not here to change your body,' my favorite SoulCycle teacher likes to say. 'You're here to change your life.'

How To Be Well

It is not uncommon to hear a forty-five-minute aerobics class described as church: many an Instagram selfie in a sports bra is tagged '#takemetochurch.' Because the meetings are so routinized, it is easy for boundaries to blur. At the height of the pandemic, my daughter asked me if my Pilates teacher, with whom I regularly Zoomed, was my very best friend.

'Ritual is so much about intention and attention and repetition,' Casper ter Kuile, who coauthored 'How We Gather,' told *Vox*. 'One of my favorite things to think about with CrossFit' — named, along with SoulCycle, as a popular millennial church alternative in the study — is that 'Christian congregations will say the Lord's Prayer at the same time every week. And here you have these workouts of the day named "the Angie," or whatever it is, and you have communities all over the world, thousands and thousands of people, doing the same ritual motion. Ritual is this really helpful way of making people think of something greater. It's a connective tissue tool. I think it also is something you can submit to in a certain way. It de-centers the individual and centers the collective in a way that I think is healthy.'

Angie Thurston, ter Kuile's coauthor, told me that when they began their research, SoulCycle was reluctant to participate for fear that it would have been a 'brand danger' to overtly associate fitness with spirituality: when Thurston and ter Kuile first invited representatives to the divinity school, they wouldn't come near it. But that changed: SoulCycle described its value as 'spiritually uplifting' in its 2015 IPO.

These days I ride alongside women in an endless parade of logo'ed tank tops that say things like 'Spiritual Gangster,' or 'Your aura is so gangster,' or 'Om namaste,' or 'Namaste all day,' or 'You are all the good things.' (Many of these come from the Spiritual Gangster brand, a company founded by two yoga teachers. Their mission statement reads like a buzzword salad: 'We are a Lifestyle brand made for and inspired by those with an unwavering commitment to the practice of high vibration living. We join ancient wisdom with contemporary culture to create elevated products for the modern wellness enthusiast and fashion lover alike. Our collections are created with intention and purpose through thoughtful design and inspiring messaging. Our goal is to create a high vibration community fueled by wellness, love, positivity and joy.')

To my great embarrassment I once, on Martin Luther King Day, rode to a disco remix of King's 'I Have a Dream' speech. 'This guy lived in the '60s,' Noa Shaw, an instructor, told us. Bearded, overweight, covered in tattoos, Noa, too, often shared stories about his struggles with addiction and obesity. 'This shit is still going on today. We need to make our bodies and our minds stronger for the fight. We need *to love ourselves, love ourselves, love ourselves.*' He told us to 'ride for the people on the buses, ride for the people beaten in the streets.' At the end of class, he instructed, 'Open your hands to accept the energy and love created in this room,' and then, on the count of three, to scream, '*Love and justice for all!*'

He shouted loudest of all and then closed his hands in prayer. 'Namaste,' he said.

And then we all shuffled out of the room.

When the pandemic closed gyms, I joined the legions of people wait-listed for a Peloton exercise bike so I could spin at home. The cultural fetish for busyness, which the Peloton founders thought they were responding to when they came up with the idea for delivering boutique-style workout classes at home, was nothing next to the need for people to locate a virtual space to share dreams, values, secrets, and hopes, and in the new era of contagion, when each heavy exhale carries the threat of ripe and germy droplets of sick, here was a community that was not bound by the need to be together physically but still provided strength and cohesion to its lonely members.

Peloton's cofounder John Foley was certainly not unaware of how important the sense of community would be when founding a fitness company in 2012. He has said, 'The stuff that happened on Sunday morning at church or synagogue is still important to human beings. It's still something humans want. But they're not getting as much of it from organized religion. People want fitness and they want something else – instructor-led, group fitness classes, replete with the candles on the altar and someone talking to you from a pulpit for 45 minutes – the parallels are uncanny. In the '70s or '80s, you'd have a cross or Star of David around your neck. Now you have a SoulCycle tank top. That's your identity, that's your community, that's your religion.'

When the pandemic arrived, Peloton was already well known for its active online communities: Working Moms, Single Dads, Pelowinos (who ride Pelotons and also drink wine), and so on. These ways of connecting became only more important as we all sheltered in place, forced to confront how, in spite of the endless virtual connection, we were ever more isolated, ever more remote. Here was comfort and community; here were charismatic leaders who addressed matters of the body and the spirit.

Years before the COVID lockdown brought communal life to a standstill, the former surgeon general Vivek Murthy described loneliness as a 'growing health epidemic,' publishing an article in the *Harvard Business Review* on the topic in 2017. In 2023, Murthy, who'd been reappointed surgeon general by President Biden, released an eighty-two-page advisory from his office titled *Our Epidemic of Loneliness and Isolation* that describes the grim health outcomes for people suffering from loneliness, which, he writes, includes more and more and more of us all the time. 'Loneliness is far more than just a bad feeling,' Murthy writes. 'It is associated with a greater risk of cardiovascular disease, dementia, stroke, depression, anxiety, and premature death. The mortality impact of being socially disconnected is similar to that caused by smoking up to 15 cigarettes a day, and even greater than that associated with obesity and physical inactivity... Loneliness and isolation represent profound threats to our health and well-being.'

Religion or not, the communal aspect of these spinning churches was, it turns out, not unrelated to the health benefits.

On Peloton, strangers are asked to ride for each other, for one member's daughter, sick with cancer and unable to leave the house. I don't know what state or even country this family was in, but I pedaled away, imagining the generated energy traveling... there?

Peloton classes are grueling, and there's something about being told, when drenched with sweat and gasping for air all alone in a garage or a guest room or a basement in the loneliness and half-light of an off-hour, even by a stranger with whom you've been maintaining only pretend eye contact for the past half hour or so, that he or she 'has got your back,' that you can do it, that things are worth fighting for, that gratitude is important, that you matter and have a place in the world. The instructor Alex Toussaint's catchphrase is 'feel good, look good, do better.' Ally Love likes to say Peloton gives you 'a crown of sweat and a soul of fire.' (It did, of course, also kill off Mr Big, which I've often thought of as I've gasped and sputtered all alone in a room.)

After the world reopened, many of Peloton's interest groups went on to meet up in the real world. The instructor Christine D'Ercole married a rider from her morning class; he was in San Francisco and she was in New York, and their first interaction was a 'shout-out' on the leaderboard.

EXERCISE

I DID NOT SEEK EXERCISE as a response to a spiritual lack in my life. I got into exercising as a teenager because I had neither the gift nor the personality for organized sports, but I was self-conscious about my body and I did not want to get fat. The first aerobics class I took was step aerobics in a little suburban strip mall while my peers chased lacrosse and soccer balls around the brown and frozen fields behind school. The instructor was Lisa; she was a young mother with enormous bangs who promised to solve muffin tops and saddlebags and not much else.

My mission has matured over the past thirty years as I have consistently stepped, Tae Bo'ed, and spun myself into a sweaty, panting state. In middle age I ask more of the practice than the straightforward slimming of my abs; I want exercise to keep me looking younger than I am, to make the insides of my body stronger and healthier and closer in form to an earlier version of myself. Like the wish of the colonic, I have often hoped that the sweat running from my pores would carry with it more than the water and salt that science tells us it does: I want it to ferry away the plain old pox not only of my banal daily agitations and stress but also of the creep of time on all the parts of me, visible and not. I've been alternately amused, embarrassed, and inspired by the wellness gospel of it all, but it's still the fitness part that keeps me coming back.

This isn't the case for everyone. Just as wellness impresarios saw the opportunity to fill a cultural vacuum by alloying spiritual pep talks with burning muscles, religious groups – mostly evangelical Christian ones – have sought to strengthen their hold on community-based spirituality by adding some wellness.

On the Apple TV show *Physical*, which chronicles the life of a fictional 1980s aerobics instructor, a Mormon real estate magnate stumbles upon an aerobics class and gasps, 'I've never seen anything like that. At least not outside of church.' It was probably a harder hit than the show's writers needed: we could see clearly what was happening in that carpeted room. The multitasking form of physical worship is, it turns out, popular no matter what you're praying to.

The current wellness trend didn't invent the idea of movement as a gateway to the spiritual self: most religions have tended to conflate the physical and the spiritual. In Christian teaching, gluttony and sloth are labeled two of the seven deadly sins, and the Buddhist belief that the mind is the body and the body is the mind is manifest in the physically grueling prostrations that Tibetan Buddhists perform and in the walking meditations practiced by Zen Buddhists. (Once I saw Lou Reed play the guitar in a sleeveless shirt. 'His arms!' my friends all said with envy. 'He's Buddhist,' I explained. I had seen a video of him performing prostrations, like so many ancient triceps push-ups.)

Catholics kneel, Jews daven, Muslims prostrate, and Sufi dervishes whirl, their continuous rhythmic motion a search for the divine and for spiritual enlightenment. Turning and turning toward truth, the dance represents a turning away from the ego in favor of truth, and then back to the world so as to be able to love fully and be of service to their fellow man. To lose oneself in music, in melody, and in rhythm has always carried with it at least a whiff of the divine.

How To Be Well

During the 1980s there was Believercise, which was sometimes called Praisercise, or Faithercise, which happened when pastors at then-emergent megachurches began suggesting an updated version of the link between physical fitness and spiritual correctness through a vast and diverse array of (for-profit) fitness products ranging from protein shakes to Jazzercise classes that remain popular to this day. The so-called prosperity gospel, also known as prosperity theology, which had been kicking around the Protestant world since the late nineteenth century, really took hold in America in the 1970s and 1980s with televangelists like Jim and Tammy Faye Bakker and is now embodied by ultrarich mega-pastors like Joel Osteen. Prosperity gospel is the simple idea that God rewards faith with prosperity and good health. Reconciliation and atonement with God are interpreted to include the alleviation of sickness and poverty, which are considered self-inflicted and imaginary, functions not of multiplying cancerous cells, let's say, or external circumstances like the race and the class one is born into, but instead of a lack of faith in oneself, a failure to think positively. Being healthy, being well, are considered signs of divine approval, so it is acceptable to worship in pursuit of not only salvation but also self-improvement and personal gain.

The emergence of fitness classes as spiritual centers is new only in the *sequence* of the combination, with exercise coming first (and without the complication of hell or damnation, except in the form of carbohydrates, gluten, and trans fat). Aerobic movement as the solution to a widespread yearning for ritual, community, music, and mission has been around for a long time.

In *Blessed*, the historian Kate Bowler offers a thorough list of pastors with side fitness hustles. 'Every major figure of the postwar healing revivals... took up [the] method of ridding the body of spiritual and physical toxins by limiting food intake,' Bowler writes. 'In fasting, believers found a porthole

Exercise

to blessings, as the process promised a leaner, healthier body, as well as new supernatural opportunities.'

In 2008, a Georgia-based pastor named Jentezen Franklin became a *New York Times* bestseller with *Fasting*, which promoted, according to Bowler, 'a whole-grain partial fast guaranteed to multiply the return on believers' prayers from thirtyfold to a hundredfold.' Pat Robertson sold 'Pat's Diet Shake,' which promised that by drinking it, you could 'lose weight, never feel hungry, improve your health, gain confidence, and brighten your outlook,' and Joel Osteen, who was a frequent attendee of Praisercise classes at his Lakewood megachurch, hosts a *Healthy Living* series on Trinity, the Christian Broadcasting Network. Pastor Paula White's *Ten Commandments of Health and Wellness* promises that 'ANYONE can do a 7 week plan that combines physical principles of exercise and nutrition with biblical references that will encourage and transform them from the inside out!' The book comes shrink-wrapped with a workout DVD in which the pastor leads the way in Lycra. Marianne Williamson, the Oprah-approved self-help guru, was best known, until she ran for the Democratic presidential nomination in 2020, for popularizing a strange and esoteric quasi-religious text called *A Course in Miracles* that she followed up with her own *Course in Weight Loss*. 'Dear God,' Williamson writes, 'Please free me from false appetites and take away my pain. Take from me my compulsive self, and show me who I am... Unchain my heart so I might live a free life at last. Amen.' And 'you don't really mean to be grasping for food. You mean to be grasping for God.'

Megachurches compete for followers with high-tech fitness facilities offering sports leagues, TRX, foam rolling, martial arts, and classes that 'mix stretching and scripture.' As the Harvest Bible Chapel in Illinois describes its Sport Ministry's goals on its recruitment website, 'Health and fitness can help build people into passionate followers of Christ.'

How To Be Well

★

The popularization of yoga in Western culture has contributed perhaps most significantly to the current state of the fitness/faith blurring. Yoga's ascension in modern America has been long, and it has been consistent. (Ignore, then, the two interviews in which Gwyneth Paltrow recounted an anecdote in which she takes credit for the increasing popularity of yoga in the United States by reminding a young receptionist at a yoga studio who'd failed to recognize her, 'Bitch, you have this job because I've done yoga before.')

Yogic tradition is thousands of years old, and its varieties and versions are vast. In the mid-nineteenth century, Henry David Thoreau found a Hindu text called *Manusmriti* in his friend Ralph Waldo Emerson's library and noted in his journal, 'I cannot read a single sentence in the book of the Hindoos without being elevated.' He put some of his readings into practice during his periods of solitude at Walden Pond, where he also read and studied the Bhagavad Gita, the basis of much yogic philosophy. And in 1893, when the Hindu monk and teacher Swami Vivekananda addressed the Parliament of Religions at the Chicago World's Fair, he introduced many Americans to the complexities of the Hindu philosophies that were contained within the practice.

The idea of separating out the physical practice of yoga for health benefits begins in America as early as 1925, when the guru Paramahansa Yogananda founded the Self-Realization Fellowship in Los Angeles to disseminate a meditation-techniques-focused Kriya Yoga practice. Another crucial figure was Indra Devi, a glamorous woman born in Latvia (née Eugenie Peterson) who escaped Bolshevik Moscow with her mother in 1917 and became an avid reader of books about yoga while studying drama in Berlin. In 1927, she sailed to India and stayed on, adopting Indra Devi as her name and becoming the first foreign woman to study with Sri Krishnamacharya, now

Exercise

remembered as the father of modern yoga. When her husband was transferred to China during World War II, Devi taught yoga classes inside the home of Madame Chiang Kai-shek. After her husband's death in 1946, Devi set sail for America, where she taught her own version of hatha yoga in Hollywood. Her version emphasized physical well-being, and her students included Gloria Swanson and Greta Garbo. Devi was, in many ways, the template for what yoga teachers would become: she offered advice on breathing techniques and discussed diet with her students, and less famous women began taking her classes in hopes of getting a little Garbo and Swanson magic for themselves.

In the 1960s, more than forty television stations syndicated a daily television program called *Yoga for Health* hosted by a handsome young yoga teacher named Richard Hittleman who had a certain genius for distilling yoga to simple, manageable movements. The show ran without interruption for four and a half years.

By the turn of the last millennium, yoga had become a mainstream exercise endeavor; fitness was booming, and spiritual seeking was ascendant. Irony had just been declared dead by the editor in chief of *Vanity Fair*, and even an editor at *The Onion* had agreed. It was suddenly okay, in the post-September 11 world, to be earnest, even in downtown New York. My colleague at *New York* magazine Vanessa Grigoriadis was a regular at Jivamukti, a fashionable yoga studio in NoHo where the hip-hop mogul Russell Simmons was legendary for his perfect plank pose. It was typical for class to begin with a short sermon, a 'setting of intentions.' The one Vanessa reported on quotes her instructor like this: "If you are a young soul, you still might be attracted to worldly offerings,' says Kelly Morris, an aristocratic-looking blonde who'd pass for a Christie's curator but for the microscopic gold stud in her nose. "But if you've been around for a couple trillion generations, the truth might be beginning to dawn that the top-of-the-line Mercedes-Benz or the younger wife is not going to do the trick for you... You always think, If I just had a promotion, I would be happier; if I just had a different boyfriend, everything would be perfect... But it never works. *More* never, ever makes you happier.'" (This is where Russell Simmons made a joke about more sex.) Later, Vanessa also quotes the instructor telling the class, 'With yoga, the reality of life will no longer be something that you have a glimpse of when you're on LSD, or when you're having an orgasm, or when someone hugs you and you have a transcendent experience and feel oneness and complete... You can have that feeling all the time.'

Yoga opened the gates, but still there persisted the idea that it adhered to ancient traditions and rituals, that yoga itself — however varied and diverse its iterations — is a valid and long-standing tradition. What the legacy of yoga has allowed is something new, communities rooted in not much at all, beyond this idea that being well has become a religion in and of itself. There is no hell, no sin, there is only the very self itself.

Yoga as practiced in the West might be devoid of its original dogmas, but the appetite for melding fitness and Christian faith seems in no danger of slowing down. SoulCore, a fitness platform that clarifies it is 'not yoga,' says that it 'integrates the prayers of the rosary with core strengthening,' with its teachers delivering instructions like 'coming up into a plank position, picture Jesus being condemned.' It saw a 50 percent increase in membership for its streaming classes during 2020, perhaps because it offered the efficiency and solace of multitasking faith and exercise. ChurchFIT, a Nashville-based fitness platform founded by a doctor named Stephaine Walker, sought to attract new members during the difficult period by reminding them, 'Had Jesus not been healthy there's no way he could have done it,' that is, carried his cross up the hill where he was crucified.

Exercise

(Walker's husband, Warren, is the senior pastor at Mount Zion Baptist Church in Nashville, and as the church's 'first lady' she is driven by a mission not unlike Michelle Obama's anti-obesity campaign.)

Some CrossFit gyms are also quite explicitly religious, in a full-circle instance of the secular going sacred. There's CrossFit Faith, 'boxes' (CrossFit franchises are referred to as boxes) that describe themselves as 'containers of transformation,' providing a space and community for accountability, healing, eulogizing, and even ritualized grieving. CrossFit Faith's motto is from the Second Epistle of Peter: 'Make every effort to supplement your faith with virtue, and virtue with knowledge, and knowledge with self-control, and self-control with steadfastness, and steadfastness with godliness, and godliness with brotherly affection, and brotherly affection with love.'

'CrossFit Faith and its members have ups and downs,' a post on CrossFit Faith's website says. 'The difference is their ability to recover quickly and move on justly. Your workout partners become your spiritual backbone holding you accountable on and off the workout floor.'

Angela Manuel Davis, a former SoulCycle instructor and motivational coach based in Los Angeles, is an Oral Roberts University alumna whose SoulCycle class included references to miracles, transformation, angels, and faith. 'My soul was tugged by the creator to take my gifts to others that were waiting,' she has said. 'In obedience, I merged movement with inspiration as I was called to do. The creator of the universe breathed life into me and created me to speak life into others. Through obedience to my call, I discovered a dynamic equation. Faith + fitness = freedom.'

I have taken spinning classes set to sermons by Nadia Bolz-Weber, a Lutheran pastor who founded a congregation called the House for All Sinners and Saints. ('Forgiveness is a big deal to Jesus. And like that guy in high school with the garage band, he talks about it, like, all the time.') And the popular Peloton instructor Ally Love, who studied theology at Fordham University, teaches a 'Sundays with Love' class that she describes as 'a spiritually grounded cycling series.' Love invites riders to call it 'church, mosque, temple… whatever feels right.' She speaks during class about moments of grace and about surrender. She sprinkles Christian music in the playlist. A typical class description reads: 'This week, Ally invites you to define humility as it applies to life both on and off the Bike. Ground yourself in sweat and spirit with uplifting musing, thought-provoking themes and spiritual inspiration in a celebration of life.' With the cadence of a revivalist she invited followers via Instagram: 'This season we will dig DEEPER, work HARDER, and explore HIGHER… we have new virtues! And it ONLY comes together if we do… so show up.'

It's maybe not the pitch I thought I was getting, but the repetition of the language makes it hard to ignore. No matter the original intention, the mission is repeated so often that it seeps in: If the stakes are that high, how dare you slack off?

SELF-LOVE

THIS LANGUAGE OF WELLNESS HAS a specific vocabulary, largely borrowed from yet another set of secular shamans, a new category of clergy that, with its bestselling books and endless stream of advice that looks catchy on social media, emerged to fill the spaces created by Instagram, podcasts, and even shelter magazines. These gurus present as the ultimate in self-realization and self-care and are somehow tolerable to the very same people who once mocked the encouraging posters that lined the offices of our high school guidance counselors: the bald eagles, the... cresting whales. Leadership. Independence. Teamwork.

Well-woman spirituality was popularized by Elizabeth Gilbert in *Eat, Pray, Love*, the 2006 memoir that details Gilbert's search for everything across Italy, India, and Indonesia. Gilbert eats pizza, wrestles with Sanskrit verse, and ultimately reaches conclusions that women should put themselves first (at least women in the financial position to chuck it all and travel) and that enlightenment, or at least peace, comes right after the gratification of her appetites.

The philosophy of self-love divorced from any nameable religion is perhaps best performed by the bestselling author, podcast host, and general wellness icon Glennon Doyle, who began her career as a self-described 'Christian mommy blogger' struggling with both alcoholism and bulimia. In the early days,

Doyle spoke openly with her followers about the ways in which church and AA were keeping her on the straight and narrow. She presented an appealing package: married to a handsome husband, mother to three healthy and beautiful kids. When she discovered, and then wrote about, her husband's infidelity, her rage took a back seat to the opportunity for self-improvement. 'The invitation in this pain,' she wrote, 'is the possibility of discovering who I really am.'

Doyle's readers joined her as she figured that out — 'we can do hard things' became her rallying cry — as she met her current partner (the Olympic gold medalist soccer player Abby Wambach) and detailed their love story, while she was promoting the release of her book. *We Can Do Hard Things* is the name of Doyle's podcast, which debuted in 2021 and made it to the No. 1 spot on Apple's Top New Shows list that year. Doyle has hosted Michelle Obama, Dolly Parton, Oprah Winfrey, Gloria Steinem, Billie Jean King, and so, so many more.

As is often the case in wellness success stories, once Doyle started 'doing hard things,' domestic bliss ensued. Doyle and Wambach now live in a much-photographed house on the beach in California that *Architectural Digest* described as 'ambrosial.' Doyle told the magazine, 'I can feel that the intention of this home is joy, love, and comfort.'

'My job is to write and feel and notice and connect and not quit,' Doyle told *Glamour* magazine in 2020. 'That's it. In order to not quit, in order to deal with being me, in order to deal with being someone who is highly sensitive, who is not just surviving, but thriving with mental differences, self-care might be my most important job.'

Brené Brown is another of these modern gurus who has popularized this language and shares a lot of views about focusing on, and forgiving, oneself. Her books, six of which were *New York Times* bestsellers, include *You Are Your Best Thing*, an essay anthology that she coedited with Tarana Burke, and *I Thought It Was Just Me (but It Isn't)* and have sold millions of copies. She is interested in vulnerability and shame, and about what happens to people who manage to cast off the shackles these feelings represent.

Brown teaches her readers that the most important thing we can do is 'own our story.' 'In a society that says put yourself last,' she has written, 'self-love and self-acceptance are almost revolutionary.' During a meeting with a group of graduate students at the University of Texas at Austin, Brown underlined the need to protect oneself: 'From the time we're born, we get feedback from people who are unskilled, starting with our parents. Are your parents all really skilled feedback-givers? We have to learn how to find the pearl. And we have to learn how to draw the line when we're being shamed.' During the pandemic, Brown hosted a few church services on Instagram. 'Unofficial,' she specified, 'I'm not a priest or a pastor.' How could anyone tell?

A newer generation of wellness messaging is different only in aesthetic. Consider the work of the poets Diego Perez (pen name: Yung Pueblo) and Cleo Wade, who often publish their work first over social media. Yung Pueblo does not use punctuation or capital letters. Cleo Wade, a glamorous personality whose daughter's nursery decor was featured in *Architectural Digest*, included handwritten notes in her book *Heart Talk: Poetic Wisdom for a Better Life*. Their messages are not much more nuanced than that 'Perseverance!' poster with the photo of the kitten dangling on a rope that stared down at me thirty years ago as I navigated my college options with a balding man in a terrible suit.

Yung Pueblo's work is often about self-acceptance: only through self-love can one heal. His poems are short enough to appear in a tidy formation in an Instagram square:

do the earth a favor
don't hide your magic.

Cleo Wade's best-known work is similarly pithy, and also steeped in notions of self-love:

baby
you are
the strongest flower
that ever grew
remember that
when the weather
changes.

The books and podcasts and social media and streaming TED talks are a new kind of pulpit; the communities they build remain largely virtual, and their followers are scattered and vast. This makes for a symbiotic relationship with IRL spaces of ritual and community: Brown and Yung Pueblo and their peers provide the gospel of confidence and self-love, while fitness and other body-wellness gurus provide the regular worship services.

The preoccupation with being 'present,' with 'noticing' and bearing witness to oneself, is especially popular in group spaces. The fitness instructor Taryn Toomey, well known for her grueling cardio program known simply as the Class, also offers 'The Course,' an online four-week 'self-study roadmap for change' through exercises, lectures, journaling, and meditation. A student testimonial on the Course website says, 'The Course has been the conduit for connecting my physical body to my spiritual being. Whereas I used to treat them independently, now I work through thoughts and feelings by spectating.' Toomey's sermons promise 'mental clearing and emotional release,' they promise eventual self-love, they invite participants to openly love themselves, to engage in 'dialogue' with their own heart.

Self-Love

'*There you are*,' Toomey prompts, clutching at her own breast. '*I'm sorry*.' She also often encourages her students to quake and scream and jump and grunt and shout and cry with their eyes opened or closed.

Of course Toomey is slim and beautiful; she wears backless unitard body stockings with tiny spaghetti straps, her long blond hair in a modified bouffant, and, sometimes, mushroom-colored knee-high suede boots with a wedge heel, which make her round, even bottom even higher, rounder, and more even. Like Gwyneth Paltrow, or Peloton's Emma Lovewell, or the pint-sized fat-free Tracy Anderson, whose perky breasts never even wiggle during her grueling dance cardio routines, these women offer a glimpse of what Anderson's disciples would like to believe is possible: success in body, mind, spirit, *and* business.

Toomey often starts class by shouting at 'the FUCKING mirror,' maintaining it's not there to look in. The real work, she insists, goes on inside the body, and she delivers a class-long monologue on the topic. It can be hard to hear over the music and the panting and the screaming and the pounding of the blood in your ears, but mostly her sermons are about self-acceptance, about the danger of comparing and despairing, about gratitude and forgiveness, primarily of oneself. Much of class is spent with hands clutching chest, saying (or screaming), 'I'm SORRY' to one's own heart.

Once I saw an acquaintance at a dinner party in Brooklyn. She had just returned from a Caribbean retreat led by Toomey. She felt, she said, amazing. 'If I can complete an exercise, which is really painful and difficult, but I get through it, then I feel like I can apply that logic to the rest of my life. I can get through anything!' she said, grinning at me beatifically. It was sloppy snowing outside and this woman was so tanned.

'And what are you up to?' she asked.

'I'm writing a book about wellness,' I said.

'Hmm,' she said calmly. 'Maybe I'll do that, too.'

How To Be Well

★

There's an increasing number of secular beauty-and-fitness-adjacent spaces to pursue this kind of language without the sweat. Sage + Sound, a wellness place on the Upper East Side cofounded by a member of the wealthy Tisch family, combines a 'nontoxic' nail salon, a café, breathwork classes, facials, massages, and a mash-up of energy work, like Reiki and sound baths and meditations. Inside, a pretty, windowless room is fitted with wraparound sofas, soft floor cushions, and blankets, and participants in the different classes are invited to settle in and relax, to listen to gonging or chanting or even silence. To hum and to yell, but mostly just to connect with their own thoughts, ideas, and sensations.

Sage + Sound also offers life coaching, which is a bit like what a member of clergy might do. The staff coach Kirat Randhawa is described as a 'contemplative guide and inspired student of Tibetan Buddhism. Her personal journey and deep course of study has led her to craft a pathway to guide others in personal development, conscious exploration, transformational practices, and life's shifts.'

While her work might be informed by Buddhist studies, this is not Buddhism. (Other classes on offer include 'manifestation,' which promises conversations on unlocking the inherent capacity within you to shape your reality.) The 'intention setting' sessions also offer 'group sharing' and 'meaningful conversations on universal themes' attractive to the fitness averse, who like the talk but not the sweat, who want to remain in a so-called wellness space, within throwing distance of a kelp salad and a guided meditation/vegan manicure.

Julie Rice and Elizabeth Cutler, two of the original founders of SoulCycle, have brought their idea full circle with the launch of Peoplehood, another company focused on classes, but these are in what Rice and Cutler have termed 'relational fitness.' The sessions are sixty minutes long and involve up to twenty strangers discussing their 'hopes and fears' in conversations facilitated by a Peoplehood guide. 'We realized,' Rice told *The New York Times*, 'that connection should be its own product.'

CULT

The Wednesday morning after the 2016 election was a day of shock and mourning in Brownstone Brooklyn, where a taco truck and a DJ had been parked, the night before, at the corner of President and Clinton Streets before sadly driving home, full of uneaten meat. That morning at SoulCycle, a teacher stood up on her altar, lit only by four large, flickering candles, and called her congregation to action. She urged us to comfort one another, to connect to our shared core values and beliefs, and told us how important it was to hold these things together. She played a lot of swooping, sweeping Coldplay anthems – movie-type music that aimed directly at the sad white liberal heart.

When that instructor left to open a dance studio called Forward Space, I started going on occasional mornings. At the end of the class was a sweaty, dark, free-form jumping, screaming moment in the dark set to self-love anthems. '*Pretty, pretty, please, don't you ever ever feel / Like you're less than fuckin' perfect*,' went one, and then: '*I open up my heart / You can love me or not / There's no such thing as sin / Let it all come right in.*' So many women screaming, crying, shouting in the dark. At the end everyone was asked to greet three strangers with an elbow bump and some eye contact, for real.

'*Go in peace.*'

At one point in my life, as I was going to about three of these types of classes in any given week, I found myself watching the documentary series *Wild Wild Country* on Netflix, about Bhagwan Shree Rajneesh and his cult's troubles in 1980s Oregon. While Taryn Toomey's disciples were not poisoning their neighbors with salmonella (the Rajneeshees did this in 1984, via restaurant salad bars), and SoulCyclers were not pledging their worldly goods to Janet Fitzgerald, there were these glaring similarities. Like Rajneeshpuram, the commune that the Bhagwan's devotees created, everything in these spaces is strongly and beautifully branded (merchandised, even) with a signature color. While the Rajneeshpuram was all about purple, burnt orange, and burgundy, everything at the Class is petal pink, ivory, and beige. SoulCycle has its own shade of sunshine yellow. Everyone in both seems a little bit high on an idea about love and acceptance and warmth toward strangers. Which, for the lost and the lonely, means it's a wonderful place to be. And then there's the jumping and shaking and release through screaming: the wild, screaming body shakes in Toomey's class are almost identical to the Rajneeshees' version of meditation, the Osho Kundalini meditation, which involves fifteen minutes of shaking ('become the shaking,' Osho instructs), followed by fifteen minutes of free dance, and then half an hour of stillness.

In both cases (both fitness and cult), the altruism is colored by ever-present consumer capitalism. At one point, Bhagwan Shree Rajneesh had ninety-three Rolls-Royces in his personal collection. Versions of the crystal talisman necklaces Toomey designs and wears and clutches during class are available in the waiting area, with four-figure price tags. Access to the supreme leader is limited; Toomey's in-person classes, for example, tend to be wait list only, so full are they of Turlingtons and Anistons and Wattses. The front row (or the 'frow') in a SoulCycle class is a place of status and recognition, much like a prominent pew in a local church. Peloton instructors shout out members celebrating important milestones. One of the effects of the democratization of fashion – all the online shopping and near-universal accessibility of goods for anyone with the cash to afford them – is that exclusivity is the hottest of commodities. These positions, attendance in these classes, having your name known by one of the status leaders, are hard-to-come-by stand-ins for logo handbags and designer shoes.

One of the fitness world's current challenges is making sure that the instructors are equipped to handle the idolatry and neediness that come with the position. CrossFit and others have struggled with sexual relationships between coaches and clients, which have long been taboo in a pastoral or psychoanalytic context, and applying these same rules in the studio setting seems appropriate because the attachment can run so deep.

'People come to class and say, "It was your voice that got me through divorce,"' Fitzgerald told me. '"It was your voice that got me to stand up and release the pain and let love into my life." Obviously, I'm very flattered and happy that people can have that experience, and hopefully I can provide a safe space for them to have their feelings, but I don't think we're ever able to really understand the capacity we have. It's probably God's way of keeping us all in check.' It's akin to a classic case of transference in psychoanalysis, but fitness instructors are not typically trained to deal with it.

'I find the guru thing hard,' Joyce Levy, a popular New York yoga instructor, told me. 'I never knew, when I became a yoga instructor, how much people were going to ask for me to be that for them. But they really, really want it, they really, really are looking for it.' It's a lot of responsibility for someone with expertise only in cardio burn rates and the correct position for a squat. The lionization of instructors is not without pitfalls: cult leaders are frequently debunked. For the Rajneeshpuram, the poisoning and the Rolls-Royces ended up putting quite a few people off. Ted Haggard, the founder and pastor of the New Life megachurch in Colorado Springs and head of the National Association of Evangelicals, was an outspoken critic of same-sex marriage when it was reported that he'd had a three-year relationship with a male escort with whom he regularly shared his massive cache of crystal meth. 'I had to expose the hypocrisy,' the escort, Mike Jones, told ABC News. John Friend, the creator of the popular Anusara style of yoga (which can be translated as 'flowing with grace'), had 600,000 students around the world (he called them his 'merry band') until losing it all in a tsunami of allegations involving sex, drugs, and money.

There's always a bit of malicious glee when someone so certain, so righteous, so clear is revealed to be a fraud. The *New York Post* couldn't get enough of 'the downfall of NYC's hottest vegan,' the tale of Sarma Melngailis, who stole $2 million from her fancy vegan and raw food restaurant called Pure Food and Wine in Gramercy Park and disappeared. Ten months later, Melngailis and her husband were tracked to a motel room in Tennessee when he ordered a Domino's pizza and order of wings using his own credit card. A couple of years later, the *New York Post* reported that she'd been sleeping with her attorney, whom she shared with El Chapo. The article included their text messages, and she was revealed to have suggested sex 'on top of the big communal table at Le Pain Quotidien' and counseled him to prepare to receive oral sex by 'eating lots of fruit and pineapple and all vegan so it tastes good.' Netflix couldn't resist. *Bad Vegan: Fame. Fraud. Fugitives* premiered in 2022.

'Hey,' I'm asked one morning outside a YogaWorks. 'Are you going to write about, like, wellness gurus who are always telling everyone to live their best lives and not eat carbs but then do lots of cocaine and sleep with other people's husbands?'

Another friend stopped me outside school pickup; she wanted to know if I'd tried a certain popular class. 'I saw that lady on the subway with her kids. She looked so tired. She was just shouting at them and, like, not even in a constructive way, just sort of shouting and guess what else?'

'They were all eating Cheetos.'

How To Be Well

★

During the summer of 2019, news broke that Stephen Ross, the majority owner of SoulCycle, was hosting a flashy, expensive fundraiser for the then president, Donald Trump, at his zillion-dollar Hamptons home. A small boycott ensued: SoulCycle was not just fitness; it was an identity. Employees were quick to separate themselves from their corporate owner, and damage control was instituted right away; in direct penance, SoulCycle hosted 'charity rides,' pledging to donate 'the equivalent of the proceeds from a sold-out class to charitable causes.' More than a million dollars wound up going to organizations like Planned Parenthood and the ACLU.

Because allegiance to a specific wellness regime suggests adherence to a set of values, to a cultural identity, because these classes often come with the promise that members are able to be more of service to their fellow citizens, instructors often make the case that participation allows one to go forth into the world in a position to help, even if it's just by virtue of the energy you're putting out into the world.

I told myself a lot of stories about the ways in which my habits needn't necessarily contradict my politics, about the many hypocrisies inherent in leading a lefty, modern, and also capitalist life, but it also revealed to me how reliant I had become on the ritual, how ingrained in my total well-being that specific mode of exercising – and its attendant affirmations – had become. I have always told myself that my relationship to exercise classes predates all the touchy-feely business, that I exercise out of some combination of vanity and anxiety. But even as I find many of the aphorisms silly and small, I have also come to appreciate the reminders about compassion and forgiveness, about kindness; to experience the release of movement without being berated about the inadequacies of my shape.

OUTSIDE OF EXERCISE

It's not just exercise. Interest in some of the calmer forms of alternative spiritualities has been on the rise, too: astrology, crystals, auras, energy... anything, really, that promises believers a connection to something bigger than themselves, an assurance that the universe has a plan. Astrology has been popular since the third century BC, when humans began to track the movements of planets in order to 'predict' the seasons. Versions of astrology have marked pretty much every society since then: with Ptolemy in ancient Egypt, through India and also China, where Confucius apparently said, 'Heaven sends down its good and evil symbols and wise men act accordingly.'

The 'hey, baby, what's your sign' of it all is a far more recent phenomenon that arguably began in 1930 when a British newspaper hired an astrologer, R. H. Naylor, to write a weekly column. Naylor had worked primarily as an assistant to a high-society self-described clairvoyant who went by the single name Cheiro and who was famous for reading the palms of both Grover Cleveland and Winston Churchill.

But Naylor soon developed a following of his own, particularly after he predicted that a British aircraft would be in trouble between October 8 and 15, 1930, and a British plane went down on October 5. So close! Close enough? Yes. Astrology's popularity has wavered since then, but according to Allied Market Research the global astrology industry is currently going bananas: it was at $2.2 billion in 2018, $12.8 billion in 2021 (thank you, COVID), and expected to rise to $22.8 billion by 2031.

It's been rejected consistently by scientists since the seventeenth century, when the study of astronomy was clearly distinguished from astrology, but as is true with apple cider vinegar, this has done little to stop it from popping up again and again and again, particularly in times of tumult and uncertainty.

The booming market is taking all sorts of modern shapes: there's Co–Star personalized astrology, which has been ranked among the top-forty lifestyle apps in the country, and there are astrology-centered dating apps (which probably work, actually, because two people willing to put up profiles on astrology dating apps are probably likely to connect, regardless of what moon rose the night of their births) and so many astrology podcasts. Chani Nicholas, Oprahmag.com's astrologer, who predicted a turbulent 2020, has seen her book, *You Were Born for This: Astrology for Radical Self-Acceptance*, through seven reprints and counting. In an interview with Nicholas for *The New York Times*, the writer Jazmine Hughes acknowledged that she should probably be more skeptical about what Nicholas said. But still, 'Ms. Nicholas's words still covered me in a sheen of being known. And being known, or at least, being treated as knowable and worth knowing, is the most comforting thing in the universe.' And as Nicholas told Hughes, 'My work – every horoscope, all of it – is just me talking to myself. I guess I need to always know that I'm not in it alone.'

The Co–Star app (which is partly powered by AI) was so popular when it launched in 2017 that it crashed from overuse three times in its first live week. It has continued to grow and grow, raising $21 million in funding over three rounds since its founding, which makes sense, because it now has thirty million registered accounts. There's also Sanctuary, which promises live chats with actual (not AI) astrologers, and the Pattern, and Chani

Nicholas's own app, and then there's Susan Miller, a New York City legend who publishes thousands and thousands of words each month for a devoted clientele who go into panic and complain mightily when she's even a few hours late with her predictions.

Crystals, another scientifically unfounded myth, are experiencing a surge, too. New York City's mayor, Eric Adams, who wears an energy-stone bracelet, attributed the city's 'special energy' to the store of rare gems and stones embedded in Manhattan schist, the bedrock upon which the island of Manhattan sits.

There have not been many conventional studies on crystals. The largest to date was done in 1999 and presented at the European Congress of Psychology in Rome. It concluded that the power of crystals is 'in the eye of the beholder.' In that study, researchers found subjects remarkably receptive to suggestion, experiencing tingling, heat, and vibrations that they were told in advance were possible. (Among the most 'suggestive adherents' to later make their way to the practice are the early- twenty-first-century reality television personalities Spencer Pratt and Heidi Montag, who spent more than $1 million of their reality show earnings on a vast crystal collection, and even welcomed their firstborn – Gunner Stone – into a birthing suite surrounded by thousands of dollars' worth of crystals. The couple soon found themselves broke and living in a property owned by Pratt's parents, but nonetheless credit the crystals with helping them to manifest a reboot of their series, *The Hills*.)

The American Queen of Crystals is Katrina Raphaell, who founded the Crystal Academy of Advanced Healing Arts in Los Angeles in 1986. Her disciples include Azalea Lee, who leads hard-to-book, hours-long crystal healing sessions in Los Angeles (Tilda Swinton, allegedly, is a fan). 'You go to some crystal shops,' Lee has said, 'and those crystals have been horribly treated from when they came out of the ground. To me, that's the equivalent of a factory-farmed chicken.'

How To Be Well

★

All of these alternative spiritualties – the boutique fitness classes, the astrological readings, the chunks of crystal lifted more gently from the ground – are an expensive way to coddle the soul. None of these institutions is nonprofit; none of these institutions is altruistic at its core. With the cost comes the expectation of some deliverable outcome, because it is their job to persuade me to come back, to spend more money on what they've got to give, to serve their investors, to serve themselves.

I will always check a horoscope if it comes across my path, and I will probably give it more credibility than I'd like to admit. I continue to exercise primarily because it has been drilled into me from a young age that in order to be a successful and attractive woman, I must be fit and I must be thin. I was weaned on *Seventeen* magazine and the diets and sit-ups described within. Consistent, punishing exercise was always described as simply part of the deal. I hope my daughters will have better ideas about things. As Angie Thurston and Casper ter Kuile's research described, exercise has lent stability in the form of ritual during difficult and isolated times. It is a meditation, even as all the rest of it is also true. I don't know that I take the magic of the studio with me into the day and spread it around, as the instructors tell us to, or even what that would mean in a practical way, but I do know that it makes me a calmer and therefore more tolerant human being.

And that I probably look better in a swimsuit than I would without it.

PART IV
PURE

It's NOT HARD TO FEEL filthy, even when you are, by most objective measures, perfectly clean: showered and laundered and trimmed, plucked, groomed, and buffed. Who knows what lurks beneath, in your nooks and your crannies? Who knows what is too microscopic to see? All the COVID in the world could fit into a single soda can.

Imagine what one entire body can hold.

In the early days of the pandemic, I washed my hands so often that my skin grew red and dry, even in the summer, when the air was sticky and wet. I backed away from friends when I met them on the street. The word 'globule' lodged in my mind, and I could picture these *globules*, cartoonish and gross, spinning in slow motion between us when we spoke. I was Carol, Julianne Moore's character in *Safe*; I was Lady Macbeth. I was those people in the desert who live in cars, cover their windows with aluminum foil, and strap antennas to their heads. If anything, I was reckless in comparison to many others: I watched a cashier's eyes go wide with panic when I opened her shop door with an uncovered hand instead of nudging it distantly with the side of my hip, in jeans I would soon throw into a scalding wash.

'Clean' though I was, I grew afraid of what lurked outside my own controllable space, frightened of the microscopic germs that could hover and leap between strangers, between friends, maybe even off *stuff*. My neighbors left their Amazon packages on the porch for days before daring to open them; they were more frightened of the murderous microbes they imagined on the goods, the box, and the tape that held them all together than they were of bad weather or thieves.

During that period I consumed news like an addict. It was too much and I knew it, but I also couldn't stop. I listened to podcasts during my daily walks, and I allowed my work to be constantly disrupted to check on this bit of news or that, which is how I grew transfixed by the story of a fifty-four-year-old man who had died of a black licorice overdose. The man was unaware that black licorice – his favorite post-work snack – contains a common additive called glycyrrhizic acid, which in large doses leads to a fatal drop in blood potassium levels. His consumption was hardly berserk: he was eating one or two packages of licorice a day at the time of his death, and he died three weeks after switching from red licorice to black. (If red licorice has a fatal breaking point, he never found out.)

In the case of this unnamed man, it wasn't the known killer slipping through a crack or a tear in a KN95 mask, or seeping beneath the sealed door of the house where I imagined he had responsibly sheltered in place. In such a wild and violent world, who would have thought to fear such an old-fashioned, comforting treat? But maybe a better question would be, who at this point wouldn't?

The scientific term 'toxins' is so overused that it now has little meaning: when it comes to the marketing of products and regimes, 'toxic' is applied to everything from relationships to odors to milk. According to even the most shallow dive into wellness marketing and reporting, there is poison in everything; no one is untouched. Death lurks in the invisible gases released from your nonorganic sheets over the toxic foam in your mattress while you sleep; poison bubbles erupt from the soap you use in an attempt to ward off all of these threats, and in the air you breathe during your meditation practice, and in the water you drink to hydrate your mitochondria after working out.

The sun is toxic (melanoma!), but so, too, are the creams you use as a shield. Not having enough sun leads to not having enough vitamin D, which leads to not being able to fight off toxins and therefore getting sick. Et cetera.

Toxins are in the fruits and vegetables you bought to be healthy, because maybe they're not quite as 'organic' as you thought, and could there be toxins in the genetically modified wheat with which you made your fancy single-batch breakfast toast? Are there dangerous antibiotics hiding in the butter you spread across it? Are your ethics polluted by the coffee with which you washed the whole debacle down? How vile is the mist from the spray bottle of citrus-scented cleanser you use to keep 'germs' from metastasizing on your countertop?

Among the earliest recorded theories about toxicity are writings by the sixteenth-century Swiss-German physician Paracelsus, who, in addition to recommending mercury as a treatment for syphilis, was an early proponent of more radical ideas about medical education. After declaring that the esteemed universities turned out too many 'high asses,' he wrote, 'a doctor must seek out old wives, gipsies, sorcerers, wandering tribes, old robbers and such outlaws and take lessons from them. A doctor must be a traveler... Knowledge is experience.'

Paracelsus's studies led him to the earliest phases of what is now the field of toxicology. 'What is there that is not poison?' he wrote. 'All things are poison and nothing is without poison; only the dose makes a thing not a poison.'

The dose.

In the hundreds of years since Paracelsus wandered Europe, the world has been flooded with new substances, but there is no real consensus about what constitutes a manageable dose of what. In excess, pretty much anything can kill you. Not just black licorice, but pineapples, apple seeds, raw cashews, water. Common sense and appetite tell us how to manage most of them. But when you are living unaware of the exposures, how can you possibly manage the dose?

One of the most common promises of the wellness industry is that it can eliminate these dangers by taking that which is 'toxic' and transforming it into that which is 'clean.' Wellness will scrub your colon, your house, your conscience. The perception of cleanliness has always counted for something in America: a turn-of-the-twentieth-century handbook for new immigrants presented personal hygiene as a successful path toward demonstrating capacity for citizenship, suggesting elimination of 'personal body odors' through bathing, use of deodorant and mouthwash, and brushing teeth. When reading a childhood favorite series of books, *All-of-a-Kind Family* (like *Little Women* but starring a family of first-generation American Jews on the Lower East Side in 1912), to my own children, I was struck by the breathless descriptions of the mother's supreme cleanliness, even in the most challenging circumstances, endlessly sending five daughters forth into America wearing spotless pinafores, ironed and pressed as a statement of values. It was the cleanliness, even more than the descriptions of blond curls on one daughter and the naming of another Charlotte, that suggested this family would assimilate well.

This old moral alignment of cleanliness and godliness, safety and sterility, has turned out to be easy to update in a world full of potential terrors, a world changing so quickly that yearning for life in its 'natural' state arises: wellness has another equally prominent theory about toxicity, however, and it can often seem at odds with purity as cleanliness.

'Nontoxic' is synonymous with 'natural,' this other line of thinking goes, in any of its commercial guises – 'raw,' 'organic,' 'unfiltered,' and so on. Even, for some, 'unvaccinated.' On one single smelly Manhattan block there is ample evidence for both schools: a Clean Market (vitamin drips, cryotherapy, infrared saunas, and CBD drinks) and a detox studio that promises 'cellular evolution' through 'gravity colon hydrotherapy,' not to mention a Skin Laundry (facials). Headlines on Goop include 'The Dirty on Getting Clean' and describe menus as full of 'Cleaned Up Comfort Foods'; wellandgood.com publishes stories like 'Yep, Your Microbiome Needs a Good Spring Cleaning, Too' and 'There's Now a Keto Cleanse for Your Face.'

Is the height of purity, then, being rid of dirt or having the *right* dirt? Antimicrobial or microbiome cultivating? A flushed colon or a fecal transplant? Cleansing or supplementing? A retreat from the pollutions of modern technology or an air purifier that looks like a spaceship?

The answer is whatever combination of all natural and all clean makes you feel better, and not (only) in the physical sense. The sphere of dangers outside ordinary control grows ever larger and more threatening: random gun violence, threats to reproductive health, climate change. Wellness operates within a very tiny sphere: your one little body in the middle of these big, menacing fears. How comforting to exert *some* level of control over the tiny little bubble of you.

CLEANSE

ALEJANDRO JUNGER, A NEW YORK City-based Uruguayan doctor, was a pioneer in the brisk business of cleansing; his 'Clean' program is at the center of his practice, and he has written five diet books with the word 'clean' in the title. Junger describes the situation like this in a Q&A with Goop:

> The air we breathe, the water we drink and shower with, the buildings we live and work in, and most of all, the foods we eat are loaded with chemicals that alone or in combination cause irritation, inflammation, sickness and, ultimately, death. Preservatives, conservatives, additives for color, smell, taste and texture, pesticides, insecticides, fertilizers, herbicides, fungicides, hormones, antibiotics, wax, chlorine, mercury, lead, arsenic, fluoride, polyhydrocarbons, DDT, PCBs, phthalates, PBA, saturated fats, trans fats, MSG, detergent and thousands of new chemicals are released every year, with thousands more awaiting FDA approval... Global toxicity is enough to overflow the body's detox capacity. Modern habits worsen the problem by keeping the detox process slow.

Junger's best-known product is a seven-day cleanse that promises to correct for at least some of that using a combination of 'intermittent fasting, Ayurveda and functional medicine to provide whole body wellness.'

Of course, it's also about getting thin. At least temporarily, and on short notice.

In 2006 a developmental biologist at the University of California, Irvine, coined the term 'obesogens' for chemical compounds that have the potential to lead to metabolic changes. These chemicals – phthalates, parabens, BPAs – are common in consumer products ranging from plastic water bottles and vinyl shower curtains to nonstick pans to sealants commonly used by dentists. Fears about BPAs do have strong grounding in science: animal testing has suggested links between BPAs and breast and prostate cancers, as well as accelerated puberty. There are also many peer-reviewed studies that suggest no discernible effects. It's a difficult effect to measure because everyone is exposed to BPAs in the course of modern life, in ways both measurable and not, so there is no effective way to isolate a control group. According to the marketing emails of any number of exciting new wellness cleanses and cures, BPAs may disrupt the normal functioning of fat cells in the body, making it harder for a person to shed weight. The FDA insists that routine levels of exposure are safe. What remains unclear is how much exposure is enough to make a difference.

Also absent from much of the marketing bonanza is whatever else such chemicals might do, which is typical of the cleanse industrial complex. With the advent of body positivity making old-school diets unfashionable, detoxification became all the more attractive as a way to envision, or at least talk about, our body goals, to continue to strive for glow. But part of the promise is still, always, to rid us of a bit of ourselves.

I first plunged into the socially acceptable world of cleansing long before I really had anything to cleanse.

Cleanse

In 2008, I was healthy and happy — thirty-two years old with a great job, healthy relatives, and a wedding to plan. But, still, I put myself on a fast. It wasn't called a fast; it was called a cleanse, which implied a higher purpose than the food skipping my friends and I communally practiced throughout adolescence. This was not my first diet — no matter how it's pitched, juicing and other dietary 'cleansing' is most certainly a diet — it was simply the first to claim weight loss as an *accidental* by-product of a larger goal, and it seemed more compatible with my phase of life and my supposed politics than some sort of calorie-restricting crash diet, which reeked of desperate adolescence and enslavement to mainstream capitalist ideas about how women are supposed to look. It was acceptable to discuss cleanses publicly because they were sold as healthy, with the lofty intent to enlighten not just your body but also your mind, and a vague association with various ascetic religious practices.

But make no mistake: the juice cleanse is a crash diet with the stink of vanity erased and the perfume of virtue in its place. I wanted to do it because I wanted to lose weight and I wanted the whites of my eyes to sparkle with health.

I chose BluePrint, which was one of the first cleansing-specific cold-pressed juice companies. Cold-pressed juices, which can sell for more than $1 for a single ounce, are the product of hydraulic presses and high-pressure processing machines. Believers describe increased value in cold-pressed juice: because pressure is used in the extraction process, no nutrients or 'live' enzymes are damaged or destroyed as the fruits and vegetables are crushed and juiced. The traditional centrifugal system for juicing generates heat that neutralizes the nutrients, they say. Less mentioned is that the cold-pressing process removes fiber from vegetables and fruits, and that juice tends to be high in sugar. Without the benefit of additional fiber, juice (cold pressed or artificial) can lead to glycemic — or blood sugar — spikes among diabetics. Especially if you're not also eating food.

How To Be Well

I picked up my coolers of unbelievably expensive juice at a loft on Manhattan's West Side in the morning as I walked to work. The juice was all I'd consume for the next three days. (One- and seven-day versions were also available, but one seemed weak and seven just seemed silly.) Even as I knew that juice was unlikely to fulfill my actual nutritional needs, it still felt like a saner and more nutritive alternative to the then-popular Master Cleanse, which was ten days of not eating any solid food, five of them consuming only warm salt water and a lemonade concoction that included maple syrup and cayenne pepper. (If followed exactly, the Master Cleanse contains about 650 calories a day – enough to stay hydrated and alive, but not much else.) The Master Cleanse, created by a nutrition guru named Stanley Burroughs, has been around since the 1940s (it was then known as the lemonade diet) and had a moment in the sun in 1976, when Burroughs published a book about it. In the 1990s, the entrepreneur Peter Glickman repackaged the diet in his own book, claiming that the cayenne pepper dilates blood vessels and breaks down mucus. The material in these books was hardly alluring: it never defines the toxins it claims to combat, but it does warn of the release of foul odors via the body and the mouth. It's unclear how Beyoncé found her way back to the diet when preparing for her role in 2006's *Dreamgirls*, but she certainly did, and she told Oprah about it, and then it was back, enough so that *Vogue*'s food critic Jeffrey Steingarten decided to try it in 2012: he described himself as woozy and weak on the diet, he describes its effect as 'ruinous' on his social life, and he vomited when he first returned to solid food. 'On the other hand,' he writes, 'I lost twelve pounds.' He concludes the article by announcing that he's definitely going to do it again.

Not long after Beyoncé revived the cleanse, I visited a friend who'd been inspired: she didn't have the energy to go outside, but she felt *great*, she said, briefly lifting her head from her creased and tangled pillow. She had started to smell a bit sour and rotten. When she did get up, she'd lost a whole pants size, which stayed away for a couple of weeks. At least on BluePrint the last drink of the day was an opaque cashew milk that had the hint, the memory, the trace of some fat.

On day 2 of my three-day cleanse, I walked to work on a bright autumn morning feeling elated: fresh, new, the world full of possibility. I felt that I had, in fact, shed something. I had risen above the pedestrian need for *food*. It was a while before I admitted to myself how closely this behavior resembled an eating disorder: I felt mostly virtuous, even as I vainly waited for the sensation of my jeans slipping loosely on my hips. The BluePrint pamphlet said there was no reason to stop exercising during a cleanse – you'll have *extra* energy! it swore – but after a three-mile run on day 3, I became so dizzy I had to lie down. My head was throbbing; my hands were shaking. I didn't feel well or clean. I just felt weak and sick. Until I gave up and ate a sandwich: I felt better right after that.

The press on all juice cleanses – not just the Master Cleanse – was quickly and remains almost uniformly bad. Juice is high in sugar, doctors warned. It strips fruits and vegetables of their natural, important dietary fiber. The body has a perfectly effective detoxification tool in the liver; avoiding food has no relationship to toxin elimination whatsoever. Juice cleanses can also cause metabolism to slow down by sending bodies into a panicked, calorie-hoarding starvation mode. This quotation, from Dr Michael Gershon, a professor at Columbia, was typical of the type of press juice cleanses got in their early days: 'The "cleanse and detoxify" idea is nonsense... The body... is not dirty inside and in need of cleansing. If you believe in evidence-based interventions, this one has no purpose. If you believe in shamanism and faith-healing, it's as good as any other form in that genre.' It never mattered: the lure of controlled deprivation was simply too great.

'It was amazing,' the BluePrint cofounder Erica Huss told me, years later. 'There would be a big piece of negative press about cleansing and we'd brace ourselves for a slowdown, but then it never came. Whatever the story, it only helped us sell more.' (Zoe Sakoutis, Huss's partner, once told me that she came up with the idea for BluePrint while on a raw food retreat where she realized that she was the only person on the retreat without a terminal diagnosis and realized that there was a market for reasons other than imminent death to seek starvation.)

The notion that you could somehow scour yourself from the inside out, rid yourself of past mistakes that build up over years, all the grudges and wounds and scars (not to mention lose weight), was simply too seductive. Those clean, cold juices were pitched to offer your beleaguered insides a rest, and with rest everything standing between you and essential peace (and those annoying seven pounds) could be washed away. Erased. Because the language around the whole thing was so earnestly presented, because it was so public and so packaged, it was easy to pretend that such vigorously controlled, restricted consumption was not just crash dieting, wasn't a deeply disordered way to think about food – much like intermittent fasting, which limits eating to specific hours of the day with a bunch of theories regarding intestinal 'rest.'

Juice cleanses got popular – popular enough that *Marie Claire* ran an article in 2013 about 'juice-orexics'; by then, BluePrint was generating $20 million in annual sales and the founders sold to Hain Celestial Group. Suddenly all the frozen yogurt joints in Manhattan turned into cold-pressed juice bars, and all of those juice bars with their white-washed walls and snappy logos were happy to 'help' customers drink juice in lieu of eating food.

Cold-pressed juice cleansing began to decline in popularity in the years after, though. By late 2015, the well-funded Organic Avenue chain, for example, which rose to meet a sudden increased demand, opening ten stores in eighteen months, had gone out of business. Five years later, BluePrint shuttered, too. This is not necessarily because of the debunking of juicing's benefits – Juice Generation, Joe & the Juice, and Juice Press all continue to thrive – but because the range of conditions considered toxic and the variety of cures available to fix them have only exploded, with juicing occupying a smaller position of an ever more crowded marketplace. Now, when I recall the bottles, I just think, *Single-use plastic? Is it even BPA free?*

Other types of cleanses are everywhere. There are raw food and plant-based meal delivery services from companies like Thistle and Sakara Life, and even the chef of New York's very expensive 11 Madison Park offers a meal subscription – a $150-per-day box for plant-based eating. There are meal replacement cleanses – ProLon, for example, in addition to Junger's twenty-one-day Clean program, in which actual food is replaced by branded supplements or food replacements. What they all have in common is that, like bloodletting, leeches, and the balancing of the humors before them, these regimens promise to make you not just a thinner but also a *better* person.

Not all cleansing procedures require full-body overhauls: there are the deep 'cleansing' breaths with which many fitness instructors begin class, and there are cleansing herbal teas, which I've desperately glugged on mornings after too much cake. There was the brief hysteria over oil pulling, which is swishing oil (palm, coconut, sesame, or sunflower) in the mouth and through the teeth for some outrageous amount of time (many suggest twenty to thirty minutes) with the promise that the oil has the power to 'pull' a variety of 'toxins' from the body, curing everything from acne to diabetes when you spit it out. (Side note: proponents of oil pulling will point to its ancient Ayurvedic roots as evidence of its power, and yes, oil pulling is a pretty effective method of low-tech oral hygiene still practiced in poor parts of rural India, where traditional practices are still widespread and access to modern dental hygiene products – toothbrushes, toothpaste, dental floss, clean water – is limited. And while oil pulling can indeed help with plaque, gingivitis, and oral bacteria, there is no evidence that it helps with any part of the body beyond the mouth. And even with regard to the mouth, brushing and flossing are, according to dentists, far more effective.)

There are digital detoxes, which can be self-administered or done on retreats featuring varying levels of luxury, but no phones. There's even been a trend of 'dopamine detox,' which requires abstaining from activities and thoughts that produce dopamine in an effort to bring the natural human drive for reward under control.

The mother of all cleanses is, of course, what I was looking for that December afternoon with Diane. If the goal of cleansing is a feeling of release or lightness, or an emptying of filth, nothing ticks all the boxes like full anal irrigation. That woman who told me her colonic made her fly – what she actually said was 'I woke up, and I was literally flying. My eyes were clear; it was the craziest feeling I have literally ever felt in my whole entire life. I felt like I *flew* all the way home' – was, she says, finally cured of a lifelong struggle with food. For years she has had colonics at least twice a week.

Colonics, which have been called 'enemas on steroids,' are used medically in preparation for medical procedures such as colonoscopies, or as a cure for extreme constipation. During a colonic, large amounts of water – up to sixteen gallons of it – are flushed through the colon via a tube inserted in the rectum. Often, a stomach massage is administered at the same time to work matter through the system, through the tube, and straight into the trash. Apart from the fact that they have no established scientific benefits, colonics carry the risk of dehydration, rectal tears and perforations, infections, and a dangerous change in electrolyte balance. They have been around since at least 1550

BC, which is when the ancient Egyptian text called the Ebers Papyrus described the benefit of an enema. At the time, it was performed sitting in a swiftly flowing river with a hollow reed inserted neatly in the butt. Louis XI had his first enema in 1480 and was so pleased by the result he ordered them to be performed regularly on his dogs. Enemas stayed popular in France: seventeenth-century Parisian society ladies often kept their own set of anal syringes, the most fashionable made from mother-of-pearl, and Louis XIV is said to have had around two thousand colonics over his life, sometimes even while receiving visitors. In the 1950s, colonics were so fashionable in boom-town Hollywood that a section of Beverly Boulevard was nicknamed Colonic Row.

Now there's Gravity, which is what I tried, which is like a high-tech, other-ended version of a gravity bong to flush away the filth. Some colonics menus offer a choice between 'rhythmic pumping action' and 'soft rhythmic pumping,' but in my experience they are much the same.

One of the method's biggest proselytizers, Gil Jacobs, a New York colonic therapist, is the insiders' colonic therapist, and he works out of a basement apartment in New York's East Village. Jacobs, who is sixty-seven years old at the time of this writing, has the skinny, haunted look of an ultramarathoner: skin taut over cheekbones, enormous white teeth. He explains the origins of his calling like this: 'I tried to kill myself because the woman I was in love with tried to marry someone else, so I poisoned myself with hydrochloric acid. I realized upon poisoning myself that I did not want to die.'

After so many nebulous descriptions of toxic states, this felt like a very specific starting point: here was someone who had ingested a known and confirmed poison, in a dose intended to kill, and then managed to heal. This was not a subjective recovery from discomfort; this was retrieval from the brink of certain doom!

How To Be Well

The story goes like this: Jacobs took himself, his changed mind, and his deteriorating body to an ER and began the long journey toward health that ends with this East Village evangelizing. 'I was deathly, deathly ill,' he said. 'I thought that was going to be it, and then someone gave me a book on alternative healing and it really sucked, but it got me into the research. I wasn't pooping, I wasn't peeing, they wanted to take my kidney out, and I had turned green in color.' Because of the book he read on alternative healing, he began getting regular colonics, washing out the poison and, with it, the sadness of his great love gone wrong.

Jacobs estimates he's had around two thousand colonics in his life and administered even more. 'Here's the belief system,' he explained. 'The only cause of sickness is retained matter unfit for human consumption. Humans by nature are gorillas, and gorillas eat fruit and leaves. The other stuff sticks in the body like cement. Beef, chicken, lamb, bread, beer, crystal meth, cocaine, sunflower seeds, tofu… when you're young you can collect and collect and you don't get sick, but when you get older and the body accumulates, you start to get sick because the system is just rotting. Dying. Picture a naked beach of eighty-year-old people: not pretty. This is where colonics come in. Let's say you're thirty and you want to live till thirty-one, you've got thirty years of dorm food, Cap'n Crunch, fluffernutter, burger platters, all the brewskis in college, maybe some ecstasy, maybe some crack. Look, the colon is meant to pass yesterday's celery, not an eleven-year-old Reuben.'

The colonic, according to Jacobs, is an exorcism, and he offers up his living, breathing self as example. 'I'm not dead, because of what I do,' he says. (He also tells me he regrew a tooth, most of which had fallen out in the suicide attempt. When I recounted this miracle to my husband, he pointed out that Jacobs had not specified where, exactly, that tooth had come in.)

Jacobs and his followers participate in a diet called food

combining, a method that has roots in Ayurveda, as well as the early twentieth-century Hay diet, and a 1940 article by an obscure doctor named Herbert M. Shelton. Food combining posits that food piles up in the intestine, causing a traffic jam effect. Shelton's followers have used the expression 'stick to your ribs' to prove their point, claiming that food might literally stick to your ribs or your gut or your colon if the right combination of foods is not eaten in the correct sequence. It's a direct inversion of most nutritional advice, which is to eat meals full of diverse nutrients, and has only ever been the subject of one scientific study, which appeared in the 2000 *International Journal of Obesity and Related Metabolic Disorders*, and that study was about weight loss, not about the buildup of 'cellular gunk.'

Food combining is not taken seriously among nutrition experts, because digestion is a complex and multilayered process. If you eat a cheeseburger, for example, digestion will begin in the mouth, where an enzyme named amylase begins to break down the carbohydrates in the bun. When the food enters the stomach, the enzyme pepsin will get to work breaking down the protein in the meat. In the small intestine, lipase goes to the fats, and on and on and on. And what about foods like quinoa, chickpeas, and nuts, which contain carbohydrates and protein and fat? To the idea of the traffic jam, Jacobs adds his own twist, which is all foods have an ionic charge, and that if you pile like upon like it will repel and shoot gleefully through your body, straight out of your butt. If, however, you combine foods with opposite charges, they will just pile up and stick there like sludge.

It's such a familiar feeling, what he describes. It's what you might feel after vacation, when you've been living on French fries and French bread and sugary alcoholic drinks with umbrellas in them: it's feeling bloated, it's feeling stuffed. But is it medically correct to imagine this traffic jam in your colon?

How To Be Well

In an ideal world, Jacobs says he would live on breath alone. It's five o'clock when I visit, and he's been irrigating intestines all day long with nary a break. I ask him what he's had to eat and drink so far that day, expecting a primer on food combining or a lecture on the merits of green juice, but the answer is nothing at all. Not even a sip of water. Aren't you hungry? I want to know. Thirsty at the very least?

'Let's pretend we're in a roomful of heroin addicts or meth heads,' he says. 'They're watching you go through your life, and at four o'clock they say, "Jesus, Amy, you haven't shot up once! That's superhuman!" But you have no heroin residue in your being. They need their poison to get through the day. It's the same with food. I haven't eaten today. I *breathe*. I'll do a vegetable juice at about 5:00, and then I'll eat when I get home, probably like five or six Haitian mangoes.'

Food, then, and even water are not life-sustaining things, not to mention pleasure, but poison: equivalent to heroin, clogging and blocking the path to bliss. They're an addiction, and an unhealthy one at that, binding you to earthly filth.

Talking to Jacobs, I couldn't help thinking of another pathology – 'orthorexia nervosa,' a term coined in a 1997 essay in *Yoga Journal* by Steven Bratman, an alternative medicine practitioner in Los Angeles, to describe an obsession with correct, or healthy, eating. The condition got a lot of attention in 2015 when a popular wellness lifestyle blogger named Jordan Younger published her memoir. Younger had followed so many diets (she was gluten-free, sugar-free, oil-free, grain-free, legume-free, plant-based raw vegan) that her skin turned orange (carrots and sweet potatoes were the only carbohydrates she consumed), she stopped menstruating, and her hair fell out in clumps. Younger describes the sensation of starving while looking for a clean option following an extreme raw food cleanse. 'What I was experiencing wasn't just run-of-the-mill hunger,' she writes, 'this was two months' worth of extreme deprivation and a week spent on purely fruits and veggies with no grains, fats, or sugar whatsoever. My body was running on zero.' Still: 'I refused to take even the tiniest bite of… pizza to hold myself over. It wasn't even an option in my mind because I was so afraid it would derail all the hard work I had put in to cleanse my system and feel good… It was my first week on a plant-based diet, and there was no way I was going to give up that light and energized feeling it gave me.'

When I told my doctor that I'd gone through with the colonic, she still couldn't accept that I'd done this by choice. She screwed up her forehead and said, 'Have you been very constipated?' as in *why the hell else would you ask?* I also asked Robin Berzin for her opinion on colonics; she visibly shuddered. 'The idea of being "clean" comes from an innate desire to rid yourself of an outside force,' she says. 'It's like, if I make the outside thing that has nothing to do with me go away, I will be okay. Thoughts can be toxic; relationships can be toxic. If you can transfer it psychologically and say I want to feel free of what burdens me and sometimes feeling physically free of something is a good proxy for feeling mentally free.'

One of Jacobs's clients had told me exactly that. Seeing Jacobs had been, for her, transformative. 'By removing the waste in my body, I broke up with my long-term boyfriend, I left my job… As I started to remove the toxicity in my body, I started to remove the toxicity in my life.'

When Jacobs looked me up and down and said, 'I could probably get five, six, seven pounds off you,' I imagined those pounds carrying with them my other, less nameable weights: anxiety, fear, stress. I pretty much stopped drinking and taking any illegal drugs after I had kids, but there I was a decade on, standing in this East Village basement wondering what it would feel like to fly home, *high*. In spite of everything I knew, I was tempted.

How To Be Well

Recently I watched a very beautiful, very thin, *very well* nutritionist post an Instagram of herself laughing on the toilet while Gil shared his wisdom beside her, eruptions and all. Her handsome husband was there, too. Gil, she said, laughing, had gone so deep. There were no secrets; there was no shame. She was emptied out of everything nasty. She farted, she laughed.

There is always the lifting of another extra layer, the expectation that only greatness is waiting to be revealed.

ENVIRONMENT

It's not difficult to get frightened by the amount of so-called chemical exposure the average person experiences in the course of a day, a week, a life. The FDA has approved more than ten thousand chemicals a year (commonly known as additives) for use in food products in the United States. (These are among the forty thousand plus chemicals in consumer products, according to the Environmental Protection Agency; only a tiny percentage of these chemicals have been tested rigorously for safety.) It does not take a chemistry degree to know that a loaf of bread that can sit on a counter, soft and unmoldy, for weeks at a time, must contain more than flour and water and salt and yeast.

It's not just what we eat, The textile industry uses about eight thousand chemicals in the process required to transform raw material into fabric, which we then use to cover our whole selves. And the fumes – so many fumes! And the water. And on and on.

Then there's microplastics, pesticides used in factory farming, air pollution caused by too many cars and Amazon trucks, and too much Freon from air conditioners cooling too many too-hot rooms. And that's before we even get to COVID and wildfire smoke dense enough to cross international borders. Many biomonitoring firms estimate that we all carry around hundreds if not thousands of synthetic chemicals in our bodies.

How To Be Well

What all of this means for your health, nobody really knows for sure. There is the question of what different 'cocktails' of these compounds might do, and what the individual response to 'body burden' – chemicals and pollutants that accumulate in a body over time – might be. Studies on the long- and short-term effects of these substances on our bodies are something of a Wild West, in part because most 'personal care products,' which include cosmetics and deodorant and hair products and soap, do not require FDA approval to be sold.

In the absence of conclusive data, and the nagging feeling that there is something enormously wrong, not to mention all the anecdotal evidence that floats about the wellness community, plenty are willing to guess and then double down. There's a great deal of speculation about the causes behind the explosion of allergies among children, fertility issues in both genders, autism, cancers, and more.

It makes sense that many of us are interested in detoxifying more than our digestive systems. Environmental wellness – a sense of security about the spaces we inhabit and the products we fill them with – is a growth industry for anyone who can afford to build a stronger bubble.

In the nineteenth century, 'filth' was considered a by-product of poverty. This was, after all, an era when untreated sewage ran freely in city streets and when minimally regulated industry released unchecked clouds of soot, smoke, and smog. To separate from filth was the ultimate luxury: wealthy people had heavy shutters, curtains, and doors. Today's 'clean' alternatives are likewise more expensive and considered higher-status: the rich now have not just water from untouched sources and virgin wheat, but also $20 aluminum-free deodorant (I can still remember a disdainful older girl in my middle school locker room watching me put on my deodorant and telling me I'd have Alzheimer's soon: these rumors are pervasive and long-standing) and $700 filters for the air in their homes.

Kobi Karp, an architect in Miami, embeds houses that he designs with sensors. 'We can use the home to get into your guts, your health, and your blood system,' he explained to *The New York Times*. Karp can install bathroom mirrors that can monitor vision changes common among diabetics; he lines floorboards with sensors for clients prone to seizures or fainting or strokes. He can install $25,000 Toto-brand toilets that can measure urine flow, blood glucose, and BMI. The company is working on its stool sampling capabilities. The article also described the efforts of a Florida entrepreneur who spent $300,000 on wellness technologies for his 8,400-square-foot Fort Lauderdale house. 'I have two young kids,' he said, 'and my wife and I wanted to give them not only an environment that is nice to live in, but also one that has the cleanest air, the cleanest water, and the right monitoring levels of toxicities. I felt a sense of security that we were moving into an environment that we could monitor.'

Michael Rubino, who describes himself as an 'indoor air quality expert and wellness advocate,' launched HomeCleanse in 2022, an indoor-air-quality company that specializes in 'mold remediation,' with both Deepak Chopra and Gwyneth Paltrow on its advisory board. 'Environmental health is the missing piece of the holistic wellness pie,' HomeCleanse's website proclaims. Rubino also claims that 75 percent of homes he has inspected have 'significant' mold or bacteria contamination. HomeCleanse offers a by-mail Mold Test, Toxic Mold Test, and Toxic Mold and Bacteria Test (the cost ranges from $274 to $724) that allow people to check for the presence of thirty-six different types of mold species in a home. 'People can't get healthy,' Rubino says, 'if they're living inside the problem.' The problem, according to Rubino, sounds familiar at this point in the wellness ecosystem. Brain fog. Chronic fatigue. Anxiety and depression. Digestive issues.

Not to mention COVID, wildfires, microplastics, pesticides from factory farming, the anxiety-fueled market for superior air. The tech company Molekule, which designs air purifiers and in 2019 was selling its flagship model for $799, was ordered the following summer to change the language in its advertising after the National Advertising Division, and a number of independent investigations, determined that the company could not scientifically or independently back up its claims, like the one that said Molekule 'destroys 3.4 million MS2 viruses in 2 minutes' or that it could ease asthma and allergy symptoms. Ultimately, it was told to relinquish its tagline 'Finally, an air purifier that actually works' and, in 2021, instructed to pay out almost $3 million in a class-action lawsuit with its customers.

In the beginning it seemed that all this regulatory legal trouble had barely caused a blip. The company attracted some new angel investors and expanded into Europe, which has been experiencing its own wave of wildfires. In May 2023, when Canadian wildfire smoke traveled south, causing the air in New York and New Jersey to turn a shocking dense shade of zombie-apocalypse orange, search-engine traffic to Molekule's website increased 6,000 percent. One New York retailer that previously sold about 7 air purifiers in a week sold 118 in a single day. Buying an expensive air purifier was something people could *do*, and even if Molekule's claims were scientifically shaky, the cost seemed to provide its own quality assurance.

Other status-telegraphing products have adapted to fit our new anxieties. The Viking, Wolf, and La Cornue gas ranges that have become conspicuous fixtures in high-end kitchens in the past decade, with price tags in the five and even six figures, are being replaced with induction ovens, which don't emit carbon monoxide, nitrous oxide, or formaldehydes. Viking and Wolf and La Cornue all scrambled to adapt their designs to match the moment – the La Cornue version starts at $15,000.

Environment

'I think at this point now, you will not find one person in the developed world that doesn't have some awareness of indoor air quality and the risks and challenges there... The learning curve has literally evaporated,' the CEO of one wellness real estate company said. Troon Pacific, a San Francisco-based building company with an expertise in 'wellness-centric high-end homes,' was installing an air-exchange system that switches out the air in a house between eight and twelve times a day.

'The better your air,' Troon's CEO, Greg Malin, likes to say, 'the better you perform as a person.'

Aside from the air we breathe, claims of pollutants invading personal space go on and on, often made from angles that allow more expensive and luxurious choices to seem obvious, ethical, and responsible. Dr Barbara Sturm, as she describes herself on her website, is 'a German doctor, orthopedics specialist, aesthetics expert and an anti-inflammatory pioneer.' Her pricey skin-care line sells $215 antipollution drops that promise to protect one's complexion from the 'often-overlooked danger of blue light from our electronic screens.' The mattress company SleepLily warns that standard mattresses might contain any or all of the toxic chemicals on the 'naughty list' it has compiled: foam made from a 'witches' brew' of petroleum-based chemicals, flame retardants, vinyl, and synthetic latex. What kind of monster would put a loved one to sleep on that? Horror stories abound: Burt's Bees, which cultivates a homey, earthy, organic vibe, was found by the FDA to have lead in one of its lipsticks. Researchers have found perfumes and colognes contain chemicals that are endocrine disrupters that can block or interfere with a body's hormones.

The cofounder of an organic cotton tampon company called Lola once told me, 'We don't want to be scare tactic-y,' by which she clearly meant that, given the facts on the table, how could they not? 'We don't want to be like what you're using is poison, because I just don't think that's building a positive relationship with the customer. It's just really about posing the question: Have you ever thought about what's in your tampon?' She then told me that conventional tampons contain an ingredient also found in common carpet cleaners. 'If they put that on your carpets, you have to leave your house all day because it's so toxic.' She told me that I was inserting that disgusting chemical in the most porous and vulnerable part of myself for four days straight, every single month. Lola advertising includes a video with a split-screen image of two tampons on fire. One burns like a match, with a crisp, defined flame. The other is melting, chaotic, grotesque. 'Conventional tampons are made with plastic... So they melt,' reads the text. The ad doesn't get any more specific, because it doesn't have to. We are conditioned enough to the horrors of toxicity that the customer can sort out which flame she'd rather invite inside herself. 'We're just trying to hit all of these duh moments,' she told me. Never once before, in my thirty-some menstruating years, had I considered that the Tampax-brand tampons I'd begun using in adolescence were doing me active harm.

Until right that very moment. And then it was like when the kids' school sends an email warning about lice: my head starts itching, and I just can't stop.

In 1962, Rachel Carson published *Silent Spring*. The book was a condemnation of the then-widespread use of the pesticide DDT, and its publication is widely accepted as the starting point of the American environmental movement. But it was also the first time many Americans began to consider what effect the rapidly developing external world was having on the more intimate landscapes of their bodies.

'Can anyone believe it is possible to lay down such a barrage of poisons on the surface of the earth without making it unfit for all life?' Carson wrote. And: 'If the Bill of Rights contains no guarantee that a citizen shall be secure against lethal poisons distributed either by private individuals or by public officials, it is surely only because our forefathers, despite their considerable wisdom and foresight, could conceive of no such problem.' And: 'When one is concerned with the mysterious and wonderful functioning of the human body, cause and effect are seldom simple and easily demonstrated relationships. They may be widely separated both in space and time. To discover the agent of disease and death depends on a patient piecing together of many seemingly distinct and unrelated facts developed through a vast amount of research in widely separated fields.'

DDT was banned in the United States ten years after the publication of *Silent Spring*. In the decades since its prohibition thousands of other chemical compounds have appeared on the market and are in widespread use, any of which contain within them the potential to harm the environment and the human body.

More than in many wellness spaces, the people at the vanguard of environmental wellness make some indisputably good points. History is riddled with examples of substances described and sold to us as basically fine (tobacco, thalidomide, the air in downtown Manhattan in the months after September 11, Johnson & Johnson baby powder, the smell of which reminds many of us of childhood but which was found to be contaminated with asbestos, which could cause a host of cancers), and so it is not ridiculous or insane to remain alert. Studies have shown how linked air quality is with overall health.

Ironically, some of the foods that have risen in popularity as a direct result of the wellness movement (quinoa, avocados, almonds) have also come with environmental hazards of their own. Quinoa, for example, which is native to the Andean highlands and contains all nine essential amino acids, has led to water shortages throughout the Andes, as well as soil erosion and a decrease in biodiversity, and with such a sudden increase in global demand production is often accompanied by low-quality practices, involving cheap pesticides and so on. The overfarming of avocados has meant deforestation in Mexico, contributing to increased carbon in the atmosphere.

Carson wrote about the rights of all citizens not to be assaulted with 'poisons' and won gains that kept DDT out of all our systems and (among other things) led to the establishment of the Environmental Protection Agency. But too many of the wellness pioneers have often contented themselves with offering bespoke solutions for the few and privileged. Asthma rates among lower-income Americans are twice as high as they are among wealthier counterparts. An eighty-five-mile stretch of land alongside the Mississippi River in Louisiana has been nicknamed Cancer Alley because of the high incidence of the disease among the mostly poor residents: in a very dark way, it all makes sense. The land there is cheap, and also home to two hundred different petrochemical plants and refineries. Cancer Alley is often cited as a prime example of environmental racism, because most of the residents of the area are Black; it is established that the health concerns of Black Americans tend to be roundly ignored and dismissed. Expensive protective technologies are not typically available in Cancer Alley, and there are no 'salt rooms' for improved breathing in the South Bronx.

While the poverty-stricken city of Flint, Michigan, wound up with drinking water laced with lead after a cost-saving measure removed the city from Detroit's water supply, a 'raw water' trend took off in more affluent parts of the country. Start-ups emerged to sell 'untreated' drinking water, claiming that processed water is stripped of valuable minerals. One brand, Live Water, was described as having a 'nice smooth mouth feel' and retails at $36.99 for a two-and-a-half-gallon jug.

ALL NATURAL

It's a long- and widely held belief that things that are man-made are more consistently 'unclean' than things that are 'natural.' It's a fundamentally conservative idea: any alterations to the so-called original nature of a thing lead inevitably to something sinister, dangerous, poisonous. Wendell Berry, a poet, essayist, and former farmer, put it this way: 'The more artificial a human environment becomes, the more the word "natural" becomes a term of value.' 'Fake,' for example, has always been the ultimate insult, whether it regards looks or character.

Economically valuable, and morally as well.

One of the clearest instances of the so-called natural preference in America right now concerns the production of wheat, which manifests itself as an increasing number of people swearing off gluten.

Gluten is a protein found in many common grains: wheat, barley, and rye, for example, which means it's present in many of the foods that many people eat every day: bread, pasta, cereal, soy sauce, and so on. A rare disease called celiac, which it is estimated affects about 1 percent of the U.S. population, is an allergy to this protein that can cause any number of gastrointestinal issues, like bloating, diarrhea, cramping, and worse. Gluten intolerance, in which more mild versions of these symptoms might appear with the consumption of gluten, is estimated to occur in about 6 percent of the U.S. population –

many of whom appear to be celebrities. Katy Perry, for example, dedicated her song 'The One That Got Away' to a pizza after her Chinese medicine practitioner told her to give it up.

But walk through any supermarket, and a massive number of products (including some that never contained gluten in the first place, like smoked salmon, peanut butter, potato chips, and even a bag of ice) are in the aisles labeled gluten-free. Several surveys in recent years have found that between 20 and 30 percent of Americans are trying to avoid gluten.

Why? Products containing gluten have been a staple of most American and European diets for centuries, without any evident disastrous effects.

But gluten anxiety comes from the simple idea that the world is changing faster than the body can adapt and evolve to accommodate these changes. Wheat has been scientifically altered to grow sturdier and bake better. We have all had to take antibiotics in our lives; antibiotics have been remarkably successful in treating and curtailing the spread of infections that used to be common causes of death, like pneumonia and diphtheria and typhoid and tuberculosis. As the rate of prescribing antibiotics for a variety of ailments has gone up, though, scientists have noted the side effect in some people of a permanent alteration in the chemistry of their guts, potentially making them less capable of managing or tolerating some foods. Without full-blown celiac disease, though, gluten is unlikely to trigger systemic inflammation, which is a condition of the autoimmune diseases that more and more people are self-diagnosing with every year.

Once again, products at the high end of the market are poised to cater to these anxieties. Einkorn, sometimes called virgin wheat, is described as the grain our ancestors ate twelve thousand years ago, long before wheat crops were hybridized for strength and durability. It costs about four times as much as regular flour.

All Natural

★

Anxiety during periods of significant scientific and cultural advancement or change is not new. This full-body, whole-self reaction has happened before, with similarly polarizing political results. In the late nineteenth century, Germany was hit hard and fast by the Industrial Revolution. In 1870, two-thirds of Germans lived rural, agricultural lives, defined by season and rainfall and whether any vermin got into the crop. Families tended to live and to stay together across generations in well-established communities. Work was physical and varied and happened outdoors.

Industrialization changed all that, with Germany having ambitions to lead, and by 1900 it had become the biggest economy in Europe. By that point, the percentage of Germans living urban lives, pursuing work in factories or mines or, in the upper classes, as engineers and architects, had increased fourfold. Suddenly a great number of Germans were separated from their families and from the seasonal rhythms of rural life. A movement called Lebensreform (life reform) coalesced, citing concerns and complaints that sound eerily familiar today: *Technology is changing the way we live! We are too far from nature! Work has become more passive and sedentary, and as a result we are less healthy. We are too disconnected from nature, from communities, and from faith.*

Medicine was advancing quickly in Germany in this same period, and just as many were challenging these advancements as well, proposing alternative solutions more rooted in nature. Christian Samuel Hahnemann proposed homeopathy, which uses natural substances like plants and minerals to encourage the body to self-heal, and Louis Kuhne opened a clinic in Leipzig advocating vegetarianism, nature walks, steam baths, and cold plunges. In Austria, the esoteric educator Rudolf Steiner began talking and writing about anthroposophy, a philosophy he invented that combined the spiritual, the physical, and the natural in pursuit of better health. A priest named Sebastian Kneipp came up with the 'Kneipp Cure,' a regimen of herbs, exercise, and regular submersion in alternating hot and cold swirling tubs. A number of Lebensreformers refused the government state-mandated smallpox vaccine.

In another presage of things to come, factory-processed food – soft white bread, for example – drew suspicion. The committed washed down dense and seedy loaves of brown bread with a nonalcoholic drink called Sinalco, which, ironically, is a sort of sugary pre-Fanta. Circulation for magazines like *Vegetarian Lookout* and *The Natural Doctor* soared, and a book by a naturopath named Friedrich Bilz advocated walking barefoot on wet grass and stones. It sold 3.5 million copies.

Frank Lipman and Danielle Claro's *The New Health Rules*, published in 2014, expands this idea that natural is best. The book contains the entry 'Wander Barefoot':

> Kick off your shoes and walk on grass, earth, or sand whenever you have the chance. Not only will this boost your immune system by exposing you to unfamiliar microbes, but it will also give you a little charge – literally. Believe it or not, just as we get vitamin D from the sun and oxygen from the air, we get electrons from the earth, which have calming and healing benefits for the whole body.

Back in Germany, the Lebensreformers splintered: some of the movement's adherents packed up their heavy bread and moved to California, opening health food stores and living in the woods. They were called the Nature Boys, and some consider them the fathers of the American hippie movement.

Another wing, also obsessed with purity, joined the Nazi Party.

POLITICS

Like a lot of things, purity is a quickly and easily politicized idea. The concept of modern life as toxic does not belong to one political position: it is fundamental to the identity of otherwise opposing sides. Gilead, the dystopic hellhole at the center of Margaret Atwood's novel *The Handmaid's Tale*, is in many ways paradisical in its wellness. The premise of the novel, and the TV show it inspired, is that an environmental disaster leads to toxicity in food, water, and air and causes a profound crisis in women's fertility and ability to bear healthy children. Gilead is the society constructed to manage the result via endlessly violent, gruesome misogyny. But also with wellness! Gilead's chief goal is a great big detox of the bodies of the fertile handmaids who adhere to a strict regimen of green juice, calisthenics, and brisk walks by the river while wearing gigantic, organic cotton petticoats. It's hardly a perfect wellness vision – there's no stress reduction, even less mindfulness – but when the handmaids shop for groceries in the gleaming Gilead market, it calls to mind Erewhon, the immaculate Los Angeles grocery chain that sells an $18 smoothie that Hailey Bieber swears is why her skin looks so good.

I sometimes wonder if the people who shop at Erewhon – with their flower crowns and electric cars – would ever browse the shop section of Alex Jones's ultra-right-wing Infowars website, where some of the same products are available, albeit in very different packaging. Ashwagandha, maca, and *Avena sativa* show up in Super Male Vitality, a supplement that 'may help support testosterone levels in men.' Ashwagandha is an evergreen shrub that grows in the Middle East, India, and parts of Africa. Powder made from the root of the shrub is said to have antioxidant, immunity-stimulant powers; it is also thought to increase testosterone in men. Crucially, it is part of a family of herbs, roots, and other plant substances considered adaptogens; *Cordyceps*, *Rhodiola*, and ginseng are others. Believers say they work as a kind of thermostat when it comes to regulating emotion. If you are stressed, they calm you down. If you are low, they lift you up. The theory finds its roots in a 1956 work by a Hungarian Canadian endocrinologist named Hans Selye whose popular theory of stress is known as the general adaptation syndrome, as interpreted by a Russian pharmacologist named Israel Brekhman in the 1960s. Selye's theory posits that the body goes through three stages when it encounters stress: fight or flight, adapting to the stress, and finally exhaustion. Brekhman's theory is that adaptogens have the power to intervene in the second phase – while the body adapts, hence the name.

Brain Force Plus is sold on Alex Jones's website because 'it's time to fight back.' The product description for Alpha Power, which contains niacin and horny goat weed, reads, 'Don't fall short on energy in the fight against power and the Deep State! Show the world what a true alpha male looks like today.' Other products include Wake Up America coffee, books on promising to reveal the truth about COVID, and Trump 'Never Surrender' T-shirts, and also superfood greens and water filtration systems.

Read blind, several of Infowars' ingredients lists are similar to those at Moon Juice, the Los Angeles wellness mecca founded by Amanda Chantal Bacon that describes its values as 'Intelligent Self Care,' elaborating that 'self-care is a revolutionary act...

Politics

We believe the first and best thing you can do for the planet starts with yourself. The world needs your clarity, capacity, and vitality now. Self-care for communal care.' Moon Juice products are covered in cosmic designs and names like Magnesi-Om, Berry Unstressing Drink, and Full Moon Sachets. Rather than unlocking a deep-state conspiracy, Amanda Chantal Bacon once told me she wishes her 'super you' vitamins had been around when she was a teenager because she might have 'gotten off the Ritalin and gotten into NYU.'

In *Doppelganger*, the Canadian writer Naomi Klein writes about the disorienting experience of being often mistaken for the American writer Naomi Wolf, whose recent political swing to the right Klein finds abhorrent. When Wolf began tweeting falsehoods about the COVID vaccine, Klein was even more disturbed at being mistaken for her.

'The world of wellness was overrepresented in a particular kind of medical misinformation during the pandemic,' Klein told *The Globe and Mail*. 'What I argue in the book is that the underlying tenets of a certain part of wellness culture are rhymed with the paranoid individualism of far-right conspiracies. The message is that you can't control the world, but you can control your body and your only real responsibility is to get your own body into a state of optimal wellness.'

One of the shadowy QAnon movement's most successful recruitment techniques is the social media accounts of widely followed wellness influencers, mixing theories about child trafficking in with recommendations for vitamin gummies and avocado shakes. It's not a tremendous stretch: because much of QAnon theory is based in paranoia, it follows that mainstream information about how best to care for oneself would be questioned and distrusted. Jacob Chansley, better known as the QAnon Shaman, who was among the insurrectionists convicted for storming the Capitol on January 6, 2021, while shirtless, wearing face paint and a big furry hat, ate organically while in prison. Canned vegetables and wild-caught tuna were, his lawyer argued successfully before a judge, central to his religious belief, which is about maintaining purity at all costs, so as to fend off external threats, both imagined and real.

The Lebensreformers who didn't become flower children gravitated into the Völkisch (nationalist, racist) movement that was later embraced by Nazi Party officials including Heinrich Himmler and Rudolf Hess. Purity, especially racial purity, after all, was a key ideal for the Nazis as well. Some Völkisch members advocated nudism for Germans: What, after all, did they have to hide? The healthy German body, they believed, was like a micro-version of the perfect white nation-state: clean and pure as the driven snow. Ernst Lehmann, a Nazi professor of botany, wrote this:

> We recognize that separating humanity from nature, from the whole of life, leads to humankind's own destruction and to the death of nations. Only through a reintegration of humanity into the whole of nature can our people be made stronger... This striving toward connectedness with the totality of life, with nature itself, a nature into which we are born, this is the deepest meaning and the true essence of National Socialist thought.

The split in perceptions of the German relationship to holistic practice presages just how pivotal a role packaging and branding can play in such a vaguely defined world. What do these things *actually* do for you, if their missions can be so easily skewed, manipulated, and sold this way or that? It can often seem that the goal is not to 'save' anyone, but simply to sell more stuff.

Speaking on the political schism over wellness, Naomi Klein

also had this to say to *The Globe and Mail*: 'We started to hear these very explicitly supremacist views, like, "Well, maybe they should die. If they don't take care of their bodies, that's not my problem." When you hear people say that, it's not such a stretch to see them in alignment with people who think people should die in the desert or drown in the Rio Grande or in the Mediterranean because they don't have citizenship. Once you start ranking human life and deciding that certain people have more of a right to live than others, you're going down a pretty ominous path.'

It's progress to consider how quickly ideas about an idealized American cleanliness are now found racist: in 2019 a New York-based health coach named Arielle Haspel (who is white) made headlines when she opened Lucky Lee's, which she billed as a 'clean' Chinese restaurant, offering variations on typically Chinese dishes that wouldn't make you feel 'bloated and icky.' Following an enormous outcry on social media (typical response, this one on Instagram from a food writer named MacKenzie Chung Fegan: 'Ohhhh I CANNOT with Lucky Lee's, this new "clean Chinese restaurant" that some white wellness blogger just opened in New York. Her blog talks about how "Chinese food is usually doused in brown sauces" and makes your eyes puffy. Lady, what?'), it went out of business in less than a year.

All that seems solid is that resistance to the pollution of modernity consistently provides a psychological buffer against the potential cruelties and random violence of life. The right practice can seem like a supportive partner, however imagined, in the us-versus-them of it all, a marker that you are more than a silent bystander in your own demise and in that of the world around you. That the choice to be well has occupied both sides of America's divided political self speaks to how pervasive the fears can be, how even peering into the rabbit hole can be enough to suck you right in.

How To Be Well

How to choose the right practice? With the right information, of course. But as we've seen, in wellness world, information and truth don't always go hand in hand.

VACCINES AND THE RABBIT HOLE

IN 2015, A FORMER INVESTMENT manager named Sophia Ruan Gushée self-published a 450-page book called *A to Z of D-Toxing: The Ultimate Guide to Reducing Our Toxic Exposures*, with chapters like 'Chemical Flame Retardants: Sons of the Tobacco Industry' and subheads like 'Arsenic in Juice Boxes.' As a reminder that government regulations aren't to be trusted, there's a long, chilling spread on asbestos. She'd been on *The Dr Oz Show*, she's a columnist at Well+Good, and she once explained to the *Today* show how to monitor your Christmas tree for creepy bugs. ('Leave the tree in the garage for a couple of days before bringing it indoors,' she suggested, 'and then shake it outdoors again. Vacuum around the tree to catch bugs and eggs and inspect the tree often.')

Gushée's obsession with toxins started when she was pregnant with her first child. She was working in distressed debt at an investment management firm at the time but staying up all night reading about how to safely raise her unborn kid.

'During pregnancy I would review every night the development of my baby,' she told me over green tea one hot summer morning. 'What I would need to eat to try and help support her development. If it was a period of brain development, I would eat extra avocados and salmon. I began to view my body as the first home of my children: the quality of my blood, the quality of the air I breathe. I approached motherhood as I did any serious job: I studied up. Every night I would review books carefully selected by pediatricians and other experts to detail what I wanted the nanny to do the next day for sleep, and diet, and play, for development. It was in that process that I started to come across information about toxic exposures. It began with learning about hormone-disrupting chemicals in baby bottles. It was so alarming to learn about this accidentally, around midnight, knowing I'd have to get up at 5:30 in the morning to start my workday, but I could not ignore what I was learning. At first I thought it couldn't be true because if it was true I would have been warned by my pediatrician or my ob-gyn or the maternity ward at the hospital, but the sources were credible. So when the financial market started to fall apart in 2009, I decided to take some time off and get control of the situation of toxic exposure in my home.'

Whatever the pressure is for a woman to purify herself, once she becomes a mother this pressure increases tenfold. The mother role is to be protector and gatekeeper: the toxins that make their way into the milk, into the home, into the air, she feels, are on her to regulate. And however much the well woman looks after herself, her ability to deliver superior wellness to her offspring is paramount. Once, as I sat in a restaurant with a well friend who was nursing her seriously bonny baby in the pretty, expensive light, she described to me what it felt like to hold a formula-fed baby. The extra weight, she said, the smell… her lip curled at the memory. What kind of mother would choose that for her child?

The essayist Eula Biss writes in her 2014 book, *On Immunity*, about disappearing down a rabbit hole of information so readily available on the internet to nervous new mothers and calling her husband in tears, insisting that they immediately purchase a new mattress for their one-year-old son. 'That morning my reading on vaccines had led me, through a meandering course, to an article about the chemicals used to plasticize plastics, which had led me to an article about the potential health hazards of plastic baby bottles, which had led me to an article about the gases released by the plastic often used to cover infant mattresses.' Compounding Biss's anxiety was another article she read about the cleanup efforts for the Deepwater Horizon oil spill in the Gulf of Mexico that involved the widespread spraying of Corexit, a dispersant that had been grandfathered into use without adequate health or safety review. Biss writes: 'I was not comforted that the oil, in some less visible form, was still roiling through the water, killing coral and sea turtles and dolphins, endangering everything from whale sharks to sea grass. In the wake of the collapse of a deregulated financial industry, I was panicked by the spillage of a poorly regulated oil industry and the leakage of an underregulated chemical industry. "If our government," I cried to my husband, "can't keep phthalates out of my baby's bedroom and parabens out of his lotion, and 210 million gallons of crude oil and 1.84 million gallons of dispersant out of the Gulf of Mexico, for the love of God, then what is it good for?"'

Biss's husband paused.

"'Let's just get a new mattress for now,' he said. "Let's start there."'

Most of the entrepreneurs and wellness fanatics I interviewed for this book talked about what they'd learned online. They have come to consider themselves experts based on the easily googleable dataverse to which we all have access, with boundaries even more unregulated than the FDA's for cosmetics. The internet is rife with rabbit holes of despair; it is easy to fall into them in the dark hours of the night, or the day, or anytime, really, because what they reveal is so fundamentally frightening.

Anti-vax sentiment has been around as long as there have been vaccines. The Lebensreformers, remember, were skeptics. When the smallpox vaccine was mandated for children in the mid-nineteenth century in England and Wales, an organized anti-vax movement blew up, one that claimed the vaccine might cause the babes to sprout little hooves and horns.

Widespread distrust among Black communities of the medical system in America has led to a distrust of vaccines, too. The perception that the medical world does not serve them and indeed dehumanizes them is compounded by the memory of the Tuskegee Study that began in 1932: 600 Black Alabama sharecroppers, 399 of them diagnosed with syphilis, were chosen for the experiment but were not told what it was about. The sick men were not offered the cure (penicillin) once it became widely available in 1943 in order for the Public Health Service to continue studying the long-term effects of the disease. The men had all been told that they were being treated for 'bad blood' and that they would be under observation for six months; the experiment went on for forty years until a front-page exposé in *The New York Times* brought it all to a halt. By then, 100 of these men had died of the disease.

Other, usually elite, communities, too, have their reasons: some of the lowest vaccination rates in the country are at Waldorf schools, schools that draw on Rudolf Steiner's anthroposophic ideas and are devoted to providing natural environments for their students, free from screens and media, and an arts-oriented curriculum. Waldorf schools describe childhood as magical and wish to preserve that magic for as long as one possibly can, to control the level of toxic influence from a world polluted by *PAW Patrol* and plastic.

The vaccine/autism panic began in 1998 when a doctor named Andrew Wakefield published a study of twelve children in the British medical journal *The Lancet* suggesting a link between the MMR vaccine and autism. That's it: one tiny, suggestive study, never corroborated by anything beyond the anecdotal, but celebrities ranging from Jenny McCarthy to Robert F. Kennedy Jr. to Donald Trump have perpetuated the notion of risk. (*The Lancet* retracted the piece, and Andrew Wakefield lost his medical license. He did, however, spend a while dating the former supermodel and current wellness entrepreneur and prominent anti-vaxxer Elle 'the Body' Macpherson after they met in 2017 at a gala in Orlando, Florida, called Doctors Who Rock.)

As one Waldorf parent wrote in an affidavit, 'I was unwilling to vaccinate because I do not believe that my child is designed by the universe/God to have poisonous substances, viruses, and other foreign substances injected into him. There is a natural and divine order in which human beings flourish, and this does not include injecting things into a human being. I have felt a sacred duty to protect my son from harm as much as possible.'

The COVID vaccine introduced a new world of anti-vaxxers to the conversation. Not about measles, or polio, or mumps specifically, but on the case of the coronavirus vaccine: during the October 2020 vice presidential debate, Kamala Harris said, regarding a potential COVID vaccine, 'If the public health professional, if Dr Fauci, if the doctors tell us to take it I'll be first in line to take it, absolutely, but if Donald Trump tells us that we should take it, I'm not takin' it.' Harris was on safe political ground here: many of her supporters felt the same way, felt that we are all on our own, we are all ultimately responsible for ourselves to figure out what in this life is out to get us, and what, exactly, we're going to do about it.

A campaign by anti-vaxxers who called themselves purebloods sprang up, and they sold merchandise imprinted 'Unmasked, Unvaxxed, Unafraid.' One self-identified pureblood wrote in a TikTok post, 'We're gonna be the antidote, because everyone else is fucked, and we're gonna be the only ones with pure blood.'

The reason people cite for refusing to vaccinate either themselves or their children is never a desire to infect other children or to revive a largely eradicated disease. It's fear.

How To Be Well

The purebloods are, of course, more likely to harm themselves and/ or others than to stay safe.

Too often, the notion that one can live in the modern world in a so-called pure state carries greater medical risk than the alternative. Too much cleansing resembles the dangers of a disordered relationship to food or to thought or to solid medical advice. In the instance of the colonic, the possibilities of dehydration and colon perforation and malnutrition and compromised metabolism are likely to be far higher than the risk of digesting supposedly 'toxic' foods in the wrong sequence. I often wonder if plugging myself with vitamins and supplements in obscene quantities is more exhausting and damaging to my body's detoxifying systems than the trace metals that I ingest.

Thinly sourced hype also threatens to become medical risk in the market for the right dirt. Antibiotic-resistant superbugs and a rise in the diagnosis of autoimmune diseases are often described as the result of neglecting the inner life, or the flora, inside our guts, creating perfect environments for bacteria to thrive. Poosh, a wellness website run by Kourtney Kardashian, suggests we 'normalize eating dirt,' specifically something called diatomaceous earth, which is 'not technically dirt… depending on how you define dirt. It's not, shall we say, dirty. Diatomaceous earth is actually of powdered fossils – or rather the fossilized remains of tiny, aquatic organisms called diatoms. Their skeletons are made of a natural substance called silica. To do the detox properly we have to consume about 2 tablespoons of diatomaceous dirt in about 16 ounces of room-temperature water. Drink the mixture on an empty stomach and at least 90 minutes before eating. This gives the particles plenty of time to set themselves up in our lower intestine before any bugs can have at your nutrients for the day.'

Katie Wells, a doula and mother of six who blogs under the name Wellness Mama, shares the steps she follows, which include allowing her children to play and crawl in dirt that hasn't been 'sprayed with chemicals,' and to put it in their mouths. Putting it in their mouths, she writes, 'is the point!'

It's a version of dirty that's *even better* than clean. Allegedly.

Fecal transplants (or 'trans*poo*sions,' as Goop calls them) are procedures in which fecal matter is transported from the colon of someone healthy into someone sick. The procedure has been around for a while and has been used primarily in the United States as treatment for a relatively rare condition called a *Clostridioides difficile* infection. For *C. diff.*, the procedure has an 80–90 percent success rate in preventing the infection from recurring. But most people don't have *C. diff.*, even if they are convinced their microbiomes are totally out of whack, which is why descriptions of the treatment have begun appearing in mainstream news outlets, like *The New York Times* ('What Is a Fecal Transplant, and Why Would I Want One?'), and on the women's fashion website Refinery29, which poses the question 'Can you make money selling your poop?' to the scientific director of OpenBiome, a nonprofit stool bank. (The FDA recently approved fecal transplants for the treatment of *C. diff.*, but also issued a warning when, in 2019, two immunocompromised patients – one with end-stage liver disease, the other with a rare blood cancer – at Massachusetts General Hospital received fecal transplants from a donor who had, among his flora, an antibiotic-resistant form of *E. coli*. One of them died as a result of the transplant.) Fecal transplants are delicate and complex procedures, even for skilled doctors, with several key variables at play. But a troubling trend had begun on social media toward the end of 2018, in which people offered how-tos on home fecal transplants, along with testimonials. 'My fatigue had lifted, gone like a storm in the night, the sky blown empty and clear,' rhapsodized someone named Carrot Quinn after giving herself two enemas using the feces of a close friend. 'I looked around me, at this brand-new world I had been born into.'

For the most part, I now find my desire for purity and control manifesting itself in less dangerous arenas. I often feel filthy for a variety of reasons: because I am aging, and the world is full of contempt for women who do. Because sometimes I eat Cheetos in an unnatural shade of red, because I just can't entirely forswear processed food.

Usually, I manage by thinking of Paracelsus and of licorice man. It's the dose, it's the dose, it's the dose. Moderation! And besides, the eager wellness woman can access any number of items harmless except to one's pocketbook.

The scalp, for example, is a whole new landscape to perfect. Where once it was enough to wash and condition hair, now there's another step: scalp purification, which requires products promising 'cold-processed' origins ('cold-processed' just sounds so refreshing), and 'water defense.'

'Defense against water before you wash your hair?' my husband said after seeing it on our bathroom shelf.

'That's right!' I answered. 'Who knows what's in that water?'

Of course, I didn't really look into what was in the water defense, either, but God, it smelled great. I wondered if it might seep into my follicles, have a go at my midwinter brain fog. And why not?

CLEANING AS RITE

However pure or natural or detoxified our scalps or colons may be, sometimes cleaning up is just good for the soul. Most major religions feature ritual washings and purification rites – various versions of handwashing, ablutions, and rebirth in water via baptisms. Wellness tends to like the word 'reset'; the theme of Goop's 2021 'In Goop Health' conference was 'Mind-Body-Soul Reset.' What, after all, is more American than a second (or a third or a fifth) chance?

In Judaism, there's been a growing movement to adapt the ancient purification rite of the mikvah, the ritual bath principally used by Orthodox women, to contemporary life, emphasizing the possibility that the mikvah can mark any important life transition. Anita Diamant, a writer who founded the Mayyim Hayyim Living Waters in Massachusetts, did so to reclaim the mikvah bath as a place and as a ritual for Jews of all types to honor life changes. And a young rabbi named Sara Luria, the founder of a modern and inclusive Jewish community space in Brooklyn called Beloved, founded ImmerseNYC, which was modeled after Mayyim Hayyim and which she describes as 'Pluralistic, Jewish, Feminist.' Luria, acknowledging the overlaps between the mikvah and the wellness process of cleansing, clarifies that there's a real difference between the mikvah bath and, say, AIRE, which is a high-end bathhouse used as a set in the wealth-porn television series *Billions*. 'The reason the mikvah works is because it's emotional. You've put in the spiritual work,' Luria says. 'I mean, I get a mani-pedi for self-care, but I don't actually *feel* better.'

Susan Goldberg, a rabbi at the Wilshire Boulevard Temple in Los Angeles (and the model for the groovy rabbi on the Amazon show *Transparent*), has found so much interest in modern mikvahs within her congregation that she's begun taking groups to Santa Monica to pray and cleanse right there in the Pacific Ocean, in the shadow of the Ferris wheel, not far from the cyclists and the skateboarders and the super-tanned old men busking with covers of the Grateful Dead.

Scientology, naturally, has its own proprietary detoxing ritual known as Purif or the Hubbard method, and it involves heat therapy, ingestion of niacin, and the drinking of a whole lot of oil and other liquids. The promise of the Hubbard method, which can last up to five weeks, is that it will clear out any illegal drugs taken earlier in life, and also that it has the positive side effect of increasing IQ up to fifteen points.

Perhaps the greatest modern evangelist of cleaning for the soul is Marie Kondo. In *The Life-Changing Magic of Tidying Up*, she describes plain old clutter as a primary obstacle to a well-and-happy life. 'From the moment you start tidying,' Kondo says, 'you will be compelled to reset your life,' and 'putting your house in order is the magic that creates a vibrant and happy life.' How can higher-level wellness exist if you can't even find a matching pair of socks?

Kondo describes a client who had invited her to stand under a waterfall. 'When you stand under a waterfall,' she writes, 'the only audible sound is the roar of water. As the cascade pummels your body, the sensation of pain soon disappears and numbness spreads. Then a sensation of heat warms you from

Cleaning as Rite

the inside out, and you enter a meditative trance. Although I had never tried this form of meditation before, the sensation it generated seemed extremely familiar. It closely resembled what I experience when I am tidying.'

(When I read this, I was reminded of the words of Joseph Pilates, the inventor of Contrology, the insanely popular exercise method that has taken on its founder's name. In *Return to Life Through Contrology*, his 1945 manifesto, Pilates describes the vitality that is released through his exercises as an 'internal shower.' He writes: 'As the spring freshets born of the heavy rains and vast masses of melting snows on mountains in the hinterlands cause rivers to swell and rush turbulently onward toward the sea, so, too, will your blood flow with renewed vigor as the direct result of your faithfully performing the Contrology [Pilates] exercises. These exercises induce the heart to pump strong and steadily with the result that the bloodstream is forced to carry and discharge more and more of the accumulated debris created by fatigue.')

When Kondo, to the delight of ironists everywhere, launched her own e-commerce site, she sold a detoxifying charcoal soap, a yuzu hand cream, and a proprietary line of home cleaning products described as 'pure, natural and unscented' and 'offer[ing] a deep clean that is free from harsh chemicals or additives.' She also began offering advice on how to 'tidy your sleep' (tip one: 'tidy your bedroom') and how to move beyond tidying to 'purify' your space. One entry on Kondo's site begins: 'Marie's philosophy of tidying goes beyond the tangible. That which we cannot see still affects us – including the air we breathe. Thus, it's important to maintain pure, cleansed energy in your space. By removing stale air from your home, you can enter into a deeper state of reflection and gratitude.' To make such happen, Kondo offers palo santo, a tuning fork, essential oils, and, as a last resort, fresh air.

Following the explosive popularity of her 2014 book, Kondo

began offering a certification program in her KonMari method, setting loose a flood of women (it is almost always women) who are ready, willing, and able to go deep on tidying as a wellness practice. In one testimonial, a Kondo client said, 'Your course taught me to see what I really need and what I don't. So I got a divorce. Now I feel much happier.' And 'I also succeeded in finally losing ten pounds.' Some of Kondo's disciples have taken note and combined their services with what used to be the purview of more traditional therapeutic counseling.

One of them, Ann Dooley, spun off the Dooley Method, which combines tidying with effective parenting. 'I used to live in a constant cycle of reorganizing our family's mess,' Dooley writes, 'feeling overwhelmed and frustrated. I resorted to yelling, bribing my kids, and blaming them for my own feelings of inadequacy. These reactive responses left me stuck and ashamed. Growing up in a cluttered home, I witnessed how it impacted my parents' relationship and influenced their parenting. It made me realize my lack of skills in creating an organized and nurturing environment for my family. I noticed a similar pattern in hiding physical clutter and my emotions of guilt, fear and shame.'

Dooley credits tidying with 'fostering creativity, calmness, and cooperation, nurturing an environment that promotes growth, happiness and lasting connections.'

It's not just parenting that can be KonMari'ed: many KonMari consultants promise that their services will improve both mental and physical health. 'Having a tidy home makes for easier cleaning and less dirt and dust buildup,' says the New York KonMari consultant Lisa Tselebidis, 'which can be the environment for germs and pests. You'll have more time for exercise and more time and money to shop for healthy foods and cook healthy homemade meals.'

Of course, it's tempting to recollect a famous quotation that is commonly (though not correctly) attributed to Albert Einstein:

Cleaning as Rite

'If a cluttered desk is a sign of a cluttered mind, of what, then, is an empty desk a sign? It's a valid question.'

But no one would ever have called Albert Einstein a well woman.

PART V
BEYOND

Does all of the aspiration of wellness have an end point? Real or imagined? Having watched the industry evolve for years, I call its ultimate promise transcendence. This takes many forms, from maintaining the jawline and ass and energy level of freshman year, to leaving this earth for a minute, to defying death itself. Sometimes it just means tripping on ketamine.

The transcendence you're pitched depends on who you are. Because wellness has become a substitution for beauty, because it encompasses the health of families and children, because strong parts of it are driven by women looking for better health options, it is largely a world of women, as this book attests. My interest in the topic is certainly inseparable from my experience as a cisgender woman attempting to figure out how to take care of myself and remain 'acceptable' in a mad, mad world.

When we get to the endgame of wellness, though, the men are out in force. They're optimizing, biohacking, expanding their minds, and cheating death and age and weakness of all kinds. Meditation, like sleep and fitness, becomes a performance enhancer. Maybe it's not so weird that we find them only now; these guys are, as they say, solutions oriented.

For women, transcendent wellness is branded as a physical and spiritual weightlessness, a peaceful stasis. It's the way you might have felt at a certain age, or even just one perfect afternoon that is seared in your memory, and you'd like to get back there. Maybe you never consciously felt that way, but it seems like something that at least should be a possibility. For some people, it might even feel like a right.

One of the more difficult concepts I've struggled with in wellness as I grow older is the notion that even though you might have missed it at the time, there was in fact one moment when you were at your best. Once you are past what society at large seems to describe as the peak age of womanhood – let's generously call it twenty-eight to thirty-five – you are endlessly sold the idea that this version of yourself has been unfairly taken away, leaving you internally sad and externally invisible. There's 'getting back to yourself' after baby; there's 'getting back to yourself' after menopause. You're always being told you'll 'feel like yourself again' when and if you lose the weight or freeze your face. Rarely, if ever, are you told you'll become acquainted with your new self, that she might be different from the old one. But of course she will be.

What are we supposed to do if not evolve, except *look* like we have not evolved?

MEDITATION / MINDFULNESS

ON A RAINY SPRING AFTERNOON, I found myself sitting in a folding chair in a fancy Chelsea art gallery clutching a deli bag full of carnations and overripe fruit, waiting for enlightenment. I was a member of a course in Transcendental Meditation, and I'd paid up to learn how to transcend using nothing more than my breath, my mind, and the mantra that I would be given once I'd offered up these gifts from the corner bodega (the registration email had contained instructions) at the makeshift shrine set up on a folding table in the very back of the room.

My teacher would be Michael Miller, a compact and smiley guy, and he was sharing anecdotes about what our future as 'self-sufficient' meditators had in store for us as we all listened and nodded quietly and supportively over the no-sound sound of the expensive heating and cooling and moisture systems that were quietly switching off and on and off and on over and over again. The gallery had been donated for the course: the owner was a graduate. *You see,* the whole thing suggested, *meditators enjoy tremendous success!*

Miller asked us to notice and flag any shifts in our behavior over the course of our four-day training. Like, maybe you'd stop cursing at people who cut you off in traffic, or maybe you wouldn't shift and sigh when the guy ahead of you on the grocery line ran back for something he forgot. *Maybe it was meditation!*

Meditation / Mindfulness

Maybe the subtle changes and shifts would be noticed by the people around you, too. Miller told the story of a meditator whose sister angrily confronted her. 'I thought you were going to tell me if you got Botox!' one sister said to the other. But of course — and here Miller giggled — of course she hadn't had Botox! Maybe it was meditation! We all laughed, of course, because Miller was telling a funny story and we were all now on the right side of smug. *Obviously* meditation couldn't smooth our wrinkles and brows. Ha! Ha-ha-ha! That's not why we're here!

But wait a minute.

No, really.

Might it?

The name of the practice — *Transcendental* Meditation — suggested that a meditation practice contained the potential to transcend our mundane circumstances, to hover above it all.

The literature on Miller's class promised this:

Reduce stress and anxiety: meditation cuts back your stress chemistry (like cortisol and adrenaline) and replaces it with natural endogenous bliss chemistry (like dopamine and serotonin).

Stay focused and clear

Meditation develops full-brain functioning. Your prefrontal cortex is activated, alpha waves increase and neurophysiology changes, so you think clearly and make good decisions.

Sleep better and have more energy

The very deep rest of meditation does two things: gives you lots of energy throughout the day and calms your system so you can fall asleep (and stay asleep!).

Be healthier and younger

Stress weakens the immune system and speeds up the aging process. Meditation reverses this: you get sick less often and you stay youthful.

Get along better with people
When you're healthier, happier and thinking clearly, you're a nicer person to be around. All your relationships get better!

Why be good when you could be *great*?
And wasn't that what meditation is for?
It's the ultimate wellness product: multiple points of entry, low potential for personal risk. It promises to make you unequivocally better, and it comes with no shortage of endorsements.

Oprah says that meditation makes her '1000% better,' Paul McCartney calls it a 'lifetime gift,' and Russell Brand, the English comedian pilloried during the #MeToo movement, says that meditation gives him 'beautiful serenity and selfless connection.' Steve Jobs was an epic meditator, and Katy Perry once told *Vogue* that meditation was a real 'game changer... neuro pathways open, a halo of lights... I just fire up!' Jennifer Aniston told PopSugar that meditation had 'really changed everything' for her. 'It's a kick start for your day,' she said, 'it centers you, your stress levels are down, and you find yourself interacting with the world much easier and better, in a calmer way. There's a peaceful joy that comes over you.' Lena Dunham started meditating at age nine to cope with her OCD. Jerry Seinfeld credits meditation for his surviving the intensity of nine years of his eponymous show ('it's like a [phone] charger for your whole body and mind!'). Halle Berry meditates, too, visualizing herself in a beautiful gazebo where her dead father tells her sweet, important things. Naomi Judd told Katie Couric that meditating was a key part of her ability to overcome hepatitis C, and Gisele Bündchen meditates with her kids. Clint Eastwood, Ellen DeGeneres, Madonna – all Transcendental Meditators.

Athletes, too. Russell Okung, formerly of the Seattle Seahawks, explained, 'Meditation is as important as lifting weights and

Meditation / Mindfulness

being out here on the field to practice. It's about quieting your mind and getting into certain states where everything outside of you doesn't matter in that moment. There are so many things telling you that you can't do something, but you take those thoughts captive, take power over them, and change them.' The Golden State Warriors announced that meditation was a big part of the reason they win so very, very much. CEOs once liked to brag in interviews how barely sleeping was key to their success; now it's all about a meditation practice. (And a good seven to eight hours of sleep, too.)

The word 'meditation' is often used interchangeably with the word 'mindfulness.' Both are so vastly and widely invoked that they can lose any meaning at all. 'Please be mindful of what you choose to flush!' says a laminated sign in a public bathroom. 'Children Who Have Mindful Parents Are Less Likely to Use Drugs or Get Depression or Anxiety,' reads a headline in a magazine I snoop on that someone is reading at a hotel during spring break.

On Amazon you can order *The Little Book of Mindfulness*, or *The Miracle of Mindfulness*, *Mindfulness for Beginners*, or *A Sloth's Guide to Mindfulness*. There's also a vast range of mindfulness workbooks and card games and coloring books, not to mention meditation cushions and the Muse 2, which is a $250 'brain-sensing headband' that tracks your brain activity, heart rate, breathing, and body movements. The Muse 2 makes it possible to 'review data, set goals and build a rewarding meditation practice.'

Goop's 'Four Keys to Mindful Parenting' instructs me on how to replace 'just brush your teeth already' with something like 'I feel angry when you do not brush your teeth and I would like you to brush them now in order to restore my trust.'

Before the pandemic temporarily shut them down, a well-funded, glamorous meditation arms race was brewing, with well-designed meditation studios staking their flags all over New York and L.A. One was James Turrell-inspired, with lighting installations. Another had a photogenic plant wall and bottomless cups of herbal tea. Yet another had a soft, tented ceiling. Walking in felt like entering a gargantuan, slightly furry dream catcher. These studios were betting on the idea that meditation would become regular and frequent and that membership to a meditation studio would be as common as membership to a gym, where the notion of caring for the mind is as familiar as exercising the body. The journalist Dan Harris, who has written two guides to meditation and hosts a popular meditation podcast, predicts that this world is only about ten years out.

The history of meditation is as vast as it is varied, containing within it scores of ideas: yoga, renunciation, the absence of a permanent self, the absence of the idea of any permanence at all, not to mention the principle of 'do no harm.' These days there are Kundalini meditation and Vipassana meditation, there is loving-kindness meditation, which offers increased compassion as a goal, and there is sound bath meditation, which is mostly about relaxation. It is possible to meditate with a guide or without, with a mantra like the one I was given (a two-syllable Sanskrit word), or your own, intention-based mantra, like 'I will accomplish my goal,' or no mantra at all. You can use meditation to wake yourself up or to slow yourself down.

Most forms of meditation have two things in common: they are concerned with the notion of mindfulness, which is, in its simplest form, the act of noticing. It is paying conscious attention to what you're doing, thinking, feeling, saying, eating, smelling, touching without passing judgment on any sensation. It is the absence of distraction: if you are fully mindful and you are tying the laces on your shoes, all you are doing for those ten or twenty seconds is tying your shoes. You are not thinking about where you might go once the shoes are tied or wondering if anyone liked your latest Instagram post about the shoes. You are simply tying your shoes, and because that is the only thing you are doing for those twenty seconds or so, you are tying the best knot you can make, but even still, the knot you tie is just the knot you tie, not better or worse than other knots out there. You can then move on to your next task with great focus and presence, occupying it fully and completely. If you have ever lost yourself in your work, or the flavor of a bite, or the sensation of lying in bed to the exclusion of everything else, you have touched the edges of mindfulness. Because the world is only ever more and more and more distracting and crowded and full, the idea of a singular focus is only ever more elusive and therefore desirable.

The second common attribute is the abandonment of judgment. The goal of most meditative projects is to experience whatever comes up without assigning it any inherent value: it just is, it is, it is.

The key figure in the uncoupling of traditional Buddhist meditation and the notion of mindfulness is a professor emeritus named Jon Kabat-Zinn, who first proposed something he called Mindfulness-Based Stress Reduction (MBSR) in 1979. Kabat-Zinn was teaching at the University of Massachusetts Medical School at the time, and he was himself a meditator; he'd started as a student after attending a talk by the Zen Buddhist Philip Kapleau in 1965.

Fourteen years later, during a meditation retreat, Kabat-Zinn had a vision. 'I saw in a flash not only a model that could be put in place,' he has said, 'but also the long-term implications.' That vision led to the idea of a secular practice that would explicitly address anxiety, depression, and other symptoms of stress via an eight-week training program. The method he taught there focused on nonjudgmental awareness, on being present for the experience without evaluation. 'I bent over backwards to structure it and find ways to speak about it that avoided as much as possible the risk of it being seen as Buddhist, new age, eastern mysticism or just plain flakey,' he said. His interest was in the possibilities of what such calm self-awareness might yield in the modern world and whom it might benefit. The mindfulness movement, he says, 'has the potential to ignite a universal or global renaissance on this planet that would put even the European and Italian Renaissance into the shade.' Also, it 'may actually be the only promise the species and the planet have for making it through the next couple hundred years.' These are bold assertions. A lot of current practices described and implemented in mainstream American wellness culture have their roots in the methodology developed by Kabat-Zinn. MBSR courses and workshops have been used by the Department of Veterans Affairs, General Mills, Goldman Sachs, Kevin Durant, and probably your mom.

What Kabat-Zinn might not have anticipated is that removing the religious connotation has not only made the practice safe for secular institutions, like public schools and large corporations, but also cleared the road for mindfulness to be a goal-oriented practice, ripe for capitalist endeavor. It is increasingly being used as such: mindfulness is sold as the ultimate performance enhancer. Or, as Arianna Huffington told me of her corporate wellness interventions, 'This is not for the people hanging out under the mango trees. Those people are fine. This is for the people who want to get things done.'

When the billionaire cofounder of Twitter Jack Dorsey revealed that he takes ten days a year to sit in silence at a Vipassana meditation retreat, similar retreats near San Francisco saw their wait lists swell. 'We are in this moment where CEOs are saying, "I'm seeing this as a really important tool that can enrich the work experience,"' said the director of development of a silent meditation retreat called Spirit Rock, where one of the teachers is the son of Jon Kabat-Zinn.

Meditation / Mindfulness

Dan Harris, the ABC News reporter, had a panic attack while delivering a live report on *Good Morning America* in 2004. He describes the event as embarrassing and painful, though I think he comes across as quite suave and professional; there's no way a viewer would know why he swiftly cuts himself off and throws back to Diane Sawyer. But it was a signal to Harris that he needed to change, and he did: he discovered meditation, and it cured him of anxiety, as well as of his tendency to self-medicate with recreational drugs (which only exacerbated his anxiety). In a perfect embodiment of the potential of the new mindfulness movement, his new self-awareness and improved mental health meant that he had the clarity and focus to, in addition to remaining a high-profile broadcast journalist, write two bestselling books (the *10% Happier* books on meditation) that begat a public speaking tour, a meditation podcast, and an app competitor to Headspace and Calm.

The rules and the boundaries for the new brand of mindful wellness are incredibly fluid: Meditate for five minutes a day or meditate for twenty. Do it in bed or in the shower or, like my friend Jenny, on the 3 express train every morning on your way to work. Go on a retreat and speak to no one for two days, or ten days, or a whole entire month if you want, or go on a retreat and speak to everyone and come home highly relaxed with a new best friend. 'Meditation: Do it,' the holistic psychiatrist Ellen Vora told Goop. 'And lower your standards for it. Demystify it. It doesn't matter if you can't clear your mind. Nobody can. That's not the goal. You simply show up for any amount of time, and then you give yourself a gold star and a pat on the back no matter what went down.' Use one of the popular meditation apps, like Headspace or Calm, both of which have been downloaded by millions of people and describe themselves as 'in mindful competition with each other.' The apps will make it easy, they'll talk you through everything ('noticing the different sounds but not getting too involved in them' and so on) and fit neatly into your schedule, but you can also close your eyes and chant to yourself or breathe to yourself. Or don't chant to yourself, just open your eyes or close your eyes. *Just. Be. Still.*

Michael Miller's journey to meditation started in college when a nice old hippie professor introduced him to the concept. 'I dabbled for a while,' Miller told me, but he also dabbled in men's rights drum circles back then. And anyway, all of that had evaporated in his adult life, which was dominated by a stressful job in corporate publishing in Los Angeles. 'I had done a lot of hippie-dippie things along the way,' he told me, 'but I just wasn't in that place anymore.'

In 2003, Miller was invited to a lecture by a friend who had recently undergone a real transformation. 'This guy,' he says of the lecturer, who was, it turns out, a Vedic meditator, 'he just had something that I wanted. I thought, if meditation is how you get that, then I will meditate. He exuded calm and happiness; he was really relatable and smart. It wasn't oobie goobie. He was like, *this is a performance enhancer.* He spoke for an hour without saying "um" or "ah"... To have that clarity intellectually is very satisfying. If it's squishy and you're smart, squishy can be not very satisfying.' Miller was satisfied. He began meditating twice a day every day right away, and now it's been fifteen years and he hasn't stopped. He even chucked his job and traveled to India to study, which is where he fell in love with the impossibly named Jillian Lavender, and they founded centers to teach Vedic meditation in London and New York.

At one point in our conversation, Miller took a napkin and a ball-point pen and began to sketch.

'There are three layers of life,' he said, dividing the napkin into sections, 'action, thinking, and being. This is where most of the wellness world is operating: action and thinking. Let's eat correctly, let's exercise well, and let's do a colonic and do all that

Meditation / Mindfulness

stuff. That's the surface level. And then there's one level down, which is thinking. Cognitive behavioral therapy, analysis, positive psychology... a lot of mindfulness exists here, what most people call meditation hangs out here. This is: let's correct the thinking so that we feel better. But then there's this bottom level of being. Consciousness awareness. That's where we go with Vedic meditation. We step beyond activity, we close the eyes, we follow the mantra down through layers of thinking, and then you step beyond thought into pure consciousness. And pure consciousness is pure. It's not possible to toxify that state. That is clean. It's stable, unchanging, creative energy. It's intelligence; it's organizing power. That's the source of it all. When you're touching that and then you move back up through thinking and action, things start to change to match what you're experiencing down here.'

I pinned the napkin to a bulletin board by my desk and found myself squinting at it a lot. What in the world was he talking about? I had nodded a lot while he was talking – it all felt as if it were making sense! – but later I wasn't so sure. What would happen in that deep, dark 'pure' state? Was this just still more talk about how to cleanse your state of being? Sometimes, there are thoughts that appear, places in the self, that are dark and unseemly, not wonderful at all. I find myself wondering about 'mindfully' committing unpleasant acts: Could I mindfully be manipulative or spiteful or just plain mean? Is the full spectrum of human emotion down there, or just the nice bits?

But if a state of pure consciousness existed, why not at least spelunk my way in its direction and see what comes up?

What Miller taught me is to close my eyes and repeat my mantra silently for twenty minutes, twice a day. That's it, that's the whole thing. Don't use an alarm to time yourself, because you will be in a state of such peace that the sound will be too harsh. You should do the first one in the morning, before you've had anything to eat. When your mind wanders (and it will wander), all you are expected to do is to notice that it has and then gently return to your mantra. If you fall asleep – head lolling, embarrassing string of drool slithering – just wake up and pick up where you left off. The main rule is to never share your mantra with anyone else or say it out loud. Because it is entirely internal, it is natural that the sound might migrate over time, but of course you will never know, because you will never tell anyone where it started or what it became.

I liked the process, particularly when I was sitting in that room, which was entirely void of distraction: our purpose in being there was to meditate, so my phone was away, my work was held at bay, my family was at home eating supper without me. I was supposed to be meditating right then and there, and so I meditated, and it was great to be so totally, completely still. Sometimes I got a weird feeling as if my jaw had separated from the rest of my face. I definitely fell asleep a few times, and I was embarrassed that this felt nicest of all. Sometimes I'd realize that I'd spent many minutes away from my mantra, like maybe even the whole time, and then I remembered to tell myself that was fine, just fine.

But finding that feeling outside that room has proved difficult, which is, of course, the point. When I told Miller that the morning meditation – which comes in the middle of packing lunches, taking showers, making breakfast, and so on – wasn't happening, he suggested I set an alarm for the quiet hour of 4:30 a.m. 'You'll go back to sleep right after!' he said, laughing a tinkly laugh. I had to stop myself from protesting that my sleep tracker goes haywire during interrupted sleep.

Nothing in the course was about anything but being a better person: it sometimes felt as though becoming a meditator meant hovering enlightened-ly above all the unenlightened assholes and jerks.

Sometimes when I'm meditating, it can feel as if the entire purpose of the exercise were just to see if I can spend twenty minutes away from checking the news on my phone, which feels like a perfectly meaningful use of time, but it's not so easily maintained. If I'm quiet at work, I can't shake the notion that someone is creeping up behind me, and I have yet to be able to detach from the sounds and, all too often, the smells on the subway train. If I'm home and being left alone (which is rare enough on its own), there's always a task to be completed, or a new episode of some very talk-of-the-town TV show to stream. (Blame my lack of meditation on HBO Max.) But since the boundaries of this version of a practice are so fluid, it can sometimes feel like permission, a guilt-free way to stare at the wall for a while, to close the door. In Dan Harris's book *Meditation for Fidgety Skeptics* he describes his wife, a reluctant meditator, finally finding a meaningful practice during the frustrating hours it took to get their toddler to go to sleep at night: this idea also made sense, meditation with the power to redeem previously wasted time. To optimize each minute of the day.

All this talk about the deliverable outcomes of meditation has put many meditation purists on edge. When I ask Miller to get specific about the 'studies' he described during my course, he sends me three papers on research conducted mostly during the 1970s; these were among the first examinations of the physical effects of meditation. One study looked at adrenocortical activity, which is to say the amount of the stress hormone cortisol secreted over a period of time. Another looked at the effects of meditation on sleep, and still another at wakefulness. In these studies, yes, it is proven true: meditation can slow the body way down, achieve brain waves similar to when we're asleep. But does this matter to the hobby meditator, to the layperson closing her eyes on the subway? Certainly proof adds to the justification of how expensive and time consuming it is to take a course on meditation.

Two of the mindfulness world's chief researchers are Daniel Goleman and Richard J. Davidson, who met at Harvard as psychology PhD students and seekers some forty years ago. In their book *Altered Traits* they describe Goleman's first encounter with Neem Karoli, known by the honorific Maharaji. He had recently become famous in the West as the guru of Ram Dass at a small ashram in the Himalayan foothills. Harvard's psychology department was just emerging from the tumult of the Leary years, and Goleman and Davidson were more interested in the possibilities of meditation than they were in the possibilities of drugs: they wanted to figure out what was actually going on in Maharaji's mind when he sat and thought for so many hours. Was his mind changing in a physical sense?

'Maharaji seemed always to be absorbed in some state of ongoing quiet rapture,' they write, 'and, paradoxically, at the same time was attentive to whoever was with him. What struck Dan was how utterly at peace and how kind Maharaji was... No matter what he was doing, he seemed to remain effortlessly in a blissful, loving space, perpetually at ease. Whatever state Maharaji was in seemed not some temporary oasis in the mind, but a lasting way of being: a trait of utter wellness.' And if his mind was actually changing into some physical state of compassion and bliss, under what terms were such changes replicable? What if we could each achieve even a portion of that? What if meditation could change not only the state of our being but the traits of our character, toward something more compassionate, selfless, and good.

But what about that 'ultimate performance enhancer' thing? What about the irony of engineers at Google using mindfulness to further addict people to the internet, for example, or the U.S. Army employing mindfulness techniques to enhance the deadly skills of a soldier? For some Buddhists, it's all just too much to bear, even when the spiritual component is *mindfully* removed from the practice. In *The Buddha Pill*, Miguel Farias and Catherine Wikholm write: 'The fact that meditation was primarily designed not to make us happier but to destroy our sense of individual

Meditation / Mindfulness

self – who we feel and think we are most of the time – is often overlooked.'

Ronald Purser, who is a professor of management studies at San Francisco State as well as a Buddhist teacher and practitioner, wrote a book about the phenomenon called *McMindfulness*, partly inspired by the unexpected collision of his two areas of interest – business management and meditation. 'It's been weaponized!' he says of meditation. 'Rather than applying mindfulness as a means to awaken individuals and organizations from the unwholesome roots of greed, ill will and delusion, it is usually being refashioned into a banal, therapeutic, self-help technique that can actually reinforce those roots.'

TRIPPING

OVER AN ELEGANT DINNER IN SoHo, a professional mentor of many years casually mentioned, as we ate our oysters mignonette, that he needed to get to sleep early. The next morning he'd be heading to midtown Manhattan for a ketamine infusion.

Ketamine, despite its reputation as a party drug, has commonly been used in ERs for decades, often for the same pain management purposes as drugs like morphine and fentanyl. In larger doses, it can produce a psychedelic experience. Sale and possession of ketamine for recreational use is illegal (it's the snorting of big amounts of 'k' in a stressful setting – like a crowded, thumping dance floor – that leaves users in the infamous 'k-hole' spiral of despair), and, while the so-called off-label use of ketamine for psychiatric treatment is largely unapproved and unregulated, it has never been banned in clinical settings, unlike psilocybin, MDMA, and LSD.

All of which means that the first medical ketamine clinics have been opening up all over the country, all racing to be established as psychedelic meccas if and when other psychedelics join the legal fold. This seems quite likely, thanks to a combination of renewed interest in the therapeutic benefits of psychedelics and a tide of controlled substance decriminalization bills that have already buoyed marijuana in many states. In the meantime, plenty of wellness lovers are eager to tune in, turn on, and get their high-performance minds blown.

Tripping

★

The Nushama Psychedelic Wellness Center is halfway up a forty-two-story Art Deco skyscraper in midtown Manhattan where other tenants include some number of dentists and so many men wearing fleece vests embroidered with the names of hedge funds, conferences, and things to do with golf. There's a Starbucks on the ground floor, fast-casual places to eat: this is worker-bee territory, and it's hard not to feel sheepish when handing over your license to the security guard and saying, 'Nushama,' to which he smirks.

Inside, Nushama is like a cross between a Venice Beach head shop and a Magnolia Bakery. Silk flowers hang in bounty from the ceiling, and the wallpaper features a pink wisteria-like pattern that is, on closer examination, clusters of fuck-bot-style digitally rendered 'nymphs,' nude-women types with tiny waists, enormous breasts, and only the merest suggestion of face. The nymphs are crawling all over each other, many in sexually suggestive positions, with their high round asses and breasts all jammed up together. There are NFTs on screens and a 'library' featuring works by Ram Dass and Michael Pollan and the Dalai Lama.

Even with all its fairly mainstream medical bona fides – the medical director was previously the in-house physician at Goldman Sachs – there's something very 'I've got a blue light in my dorm room' about the whole place, even as competent-looking nurses in scrubs bustle among the eighteen treatment rooms where 'members' undertake their journeys in zero-gravity lounge chairs while listening to a carefully curated soundtrack that includes 'Here Comes the Sun.'

Its mission statement reads: 'Our goal is to inspire you to transform your life and to provide a sanctuary to support you as you embark on your mental health journey. We built our wellness center with this in mind, weaving nature and art into every room to evoke a childlike sense of wonder and help foster a deeper connection to the healing power within all of us.'

Nushama was born when a fashion designer with a side interest in 'plant medicine' named Jay Godfrey began to lose his business during the early days of the pandemic. He read the journalist Michael Pollan's bestselling 2018 book on psychedelics, *How to Change Your Mind*; he traveled to Mexico and participated in a substance-aided 'journey,' partly inspired by Pollan's book. When he got back to New York, he found that he was taking the end of his career in perfect stride. 'I just wasn't upset,' he says, 'and I really should have been.' He attributed this equilibrium to the drugs.

Godfrey was then introduced by mutual friends to Steven Radowitz, an internal medicine physician with a deep interest in the spiritual. A longtime follower of Kabbalah – or Jewish mysticism – Radowitz was intrigued by the mind-changing possibilities of ketamine, the connection between health and something less tangible, something divine. Ketamine, they both felt, has the power to melt the ego away, leaving the patient in touch with her deepest truths, able to confront them without judgment. The goals are not unlike those of meditation or of psychoanalysis; they are more like a turbocharged version of both, accessible via IV, attainable in six sessions.

Wellness being considered a part of the counterculture has often worked against some of its more promising notions. As Pollan writes in *How to Change Your Mind,* an NYU researcher named Stephen Ross discovered that psychedelics had been widely used during the 1950s to treat addiction, depression, OCD, schizophrenia, autism, and end-of-life anxiety. 'There had been forty thousand research participants,' Ross told Pollan, 'and more than a thousand clinical papers! The American Psychiatric Association had whole meetings centered around LSD, this new wonder drug. Some of the best minds in psychiatry had seriously studied these compounds in therapeutic models, with government funding.'

But then. Timothy Leary and his colleague Richard Alpert (known as Ram Dass) launched the Harvard Psilocybin Project and set off one of the great moral panics of the twentieth century when their research went off the academic rails. They were shut down and discredited when their experimentation began to seem as recreational as it was scientific. There is a story about President Richard Nixon calling Leary 'the most dangerous man in America,' and although it's unclear if he ever did say this, the schism between this kind of medical experimentation and the establishment was strong enough that the story is widely believed and repeated. In 1968, LSD was banned in America, and the passage of the Controlled Substances Act in 1970 meant that research into psilocybins would have to immediately stop, and with it a major area of inquiry into how we, as humans, might become what Halbert Dunn described: better than well.

It is not that this type of seeking stopped, but it definitively separated from the mainstream. Meditation centers, psychedelic drugs, meditators, and so on were countercultural epicenters of nudity, long hair, physical manifestations of Leary's suggestion that young people 'turn on, tune in, drop out.' Dropping out implied a separation from striving society, a far cry from the optimized notion of 'winning' that these modes of exploration certainly promise now. To participate in them was to separate oneself from the dominant culture, and it was as political and rebellious a statement as anything else.

It would be hard for Timothy Leary to imagine our current CBD state, where janky-looking storefronts offer a variety of CBD options ranging from the medical to the purely recreational. (CBD is, put simply, the non-psychoactive portion of the marijuana or hemp plant. The idea is that, once separated from its psychoactive properties, CBD has the potential to safely and neutrally treat the exact kind of buffet of symptoms that wellness fixes often promise to cure: everything from brain fog to inflammation to more generalized notions of performance.) Far from looking like opportunities to drop out, CBD is more often marketed as the ultimate means of 'plugging in.' An NIH study found that CBD could increase oxygen consumption and pleasure ratings during endurance running, and even protect against myocardial injury. A million clinical trials are looking into the relationship between CBD and anxiety, insomnia, and chronic pain, while a million start-ups sell gummies and vape pens and products that play with the ratio of CBD to THC (the psychoactive part of the plant). *The New York Times* described CBD as having the potential to 'provide a kind of full-body massage at the molecular level,' and maybe even bring the entire symphony that is the human brain into harmony.

But CBD has largely stalled. Laws are still too varied, and products are wildly inconsistent. More popular is good old-fashioned getting stoned, it seems, or even undergoing the wild ritual of an ayahuasca ceremony, complete with vomiting and visions and emerging better equipped to take on the world.

I spent a while flirting with the idea of trying ketamine, but ultimately I chickened out. It was a few things: it was the wallpaper at Nushama (I wanted to believe the medical side of things, but ultimately just couldn't take men who claimed to treat eating disorders with fuck-bots on the wallpaper seriously). It was Matthew Perry dying with all that ketamine in his blood. It was my Gen X relationship to the term 'k-hole.' It was my friend who couldn't get her heart rate below 95 for months after completing her therapy.

WHAT ABOUT MEN?

This is a book about women, because this is an industry about women in a world that has disproportionately placed the burden of being healthy and attractive on us. I've often been struck by the cluelessness of intelligent, educated men when it comes to matters of physical self-improvement. My brother was shocked by his weight gain in his freshman year at college, so I asked him to describe what he was eating. It was the easiest sisterly advice I've ever given: I told him if he just drank water instead of Diet Dr Pepper he'd probably be fine. (It worked.) When I met my husband, he was baffled by my knowledge of diets and exercise and skin-care regimes, and even more baffled when I explained that any woman with a casual, waiting-room-and-nail-salon relationship to women's magazines knew just as much as, if not more than, I do about the endless utility of almonds.

Most wellness gyms, spas, and other protocols describe a clientele that skews about eighty-twenty female to male. There is evidence for this position. American women tend to outlive American men by nearly six years (a male baby born in 2021 has an average life expectancy of 73.5, while his sister can expect to make it to 79.3), and women even found themselves less likely to suffer from COVID. It might be because women are so well conditioned to attempt improvement in their physical appearance. At my twenty-fifth college reunion, the women all looked younger than the men: carefully colored hair, carefully applied makeup, figures toned by exercise regimens we've been honing since our senior years, if not earlier. The men were often balder, paunchier, and seemingly unbothered by it.

Women are sold the 'body after baby!' success stories, and meanwhile men get 'dad bod,' an expression that took off in 2015 after a Clemson University student named Mackenzie Pearson wrote an article on the phenomenon that observed, 'While we all love a sculpted guy, there is just something about the dad bod that makes boys seem more human, natural, and attractive.' The article was soon followed by a 'flow chart' in *The Washington Post* that used a somewhat subjective BMI-based chart to conclude that there are more 'dad bods' in the United States than there are people in Australia, and *GQ* offered this: 'As long as you're not taking dad bod to Depardieu territory, you're golden. No shame in having a dad bod or being comfortable in your own skin. Dads fucking rule!'

In June 2019, *The New York Times* published an op-ed by the novelist Jessica Knoll called 'Smash the Wellness Industry.' 'Why are so many smart women falling for its harmful, pseudoscientific claims?' was the subhead, and in the piece Knoll described sitting down to a business lunch in Los Angeles with a group of accomplished women who immediately launched into lamentations on the failings of their bodies and of their own failures to follow strict 'wellness' guidelines to better bodies and better lives. Knoll glances around the restaurant at the men tucking into their cheeseburgers. 'When men sit down to a business lunch, they don't waste it pointing out every flaw on their bodies. They discuss ideas, strategies, their plans to take up more space than they already do.'

But what *about* men?

Things may be – slowly – changing. My twenty-fifth reunion peers and I are of a generation that excused the appearance of men, particularly if their money and status were secure. This is no longer such a given: men are an increasing and tempting market, not least because social media and dating apps have both subjected the male body to an unprecedented amount of scrutiny. Bulging biceps and washboard abs, something called the 'Dorito physique' on TikTok (not because you eat them, but because you are shaped like one, with huge shoulders and a tiny waist), get results and responses on those platforms, and many young (and some not-so-young) men are feeling the pressure to pump up. In its extreme manifestation, the desire has been called bigorexia.

This qualifies as a relatively recent trend only for straight, cis men and teenagers, it should be said. A lot of modern American gym culture is an outgrowth and appropriation of the gay gym culture that flourished in New York, San Francisco, and Los Angeles during the 1970s and 1980s, when sex-segregated gyms were uniquely safe spaces where men could be out, could flaunt, flirt, admire, and meet. This changed with the arrival of the AIDS epidemic, when gyms remained places to keep doing all that, but also became places to instruct and learn how to take care of bodies both sick and well and to demonstrate the strength and well-being of the uninfected. Once AIDS became treatable, physical fitness became a piece of the cocktail of drugs and therapies that were helping to control and contain the disease. Today, the desire for a muscly, gym-buffed body flourishes across sexual identities, often sans knowledge of its history.

Often, when men did pursue female-style 'wellness' endeavors, they were mocked not as female but as effete. The 1990s term 'metrosexual,' which referred to urban dandies who liked hair gel and rare Japanese denim and generally preferred women for sex, had homophobic implications in its very name. The irony of straight-man wellness culture's debt to gay gym culture is, naturally, unacknowledged. A men's makeup brand that launched in 2019 adopted the dubious name

War Paint and an ad campaign that so aggressively asserted its hetero-masculinity – skull rings, hand tattoos, enormous pecs, a partnership with the Wigan Warriors rugby team – that it reads more like camp.

Hims was heralded as the first big men's wellness company when it was founded in 2017. (At the time of this writing, its market valuation is $1.9 billion.) It launched with an aggressive advertising campaign in New York City. Every subway car was awash in Hims beige, pink, bright white bleeding to the edges of the posters, a single fiddlehead fern here, stark black type there, and lots of fresh-faced young men of many races wearing clean white T-shirts and horn-rimmed glasses, smiling with optic-white symmetric teeth. One ad featured the strong, proud bell-shaped end of a cactus plant. In another, a feminine, manicured hand gripped a banana. If you followed the ad's directions to the forhims.com website, you'd get the following greeting: 'Guy, Against staggering odds two things happened. One, the universe. Two, you. Let's walk at our full height, honor the forebears, have a smile and for god's sake, floss.'

Hims was the brainchild of Andrew Dudum, a twenty-nine-year-old from San Francisco who had the idea for the business when his sisters complained that his skin was 'ashy.' 'Like, I'm a guy,' he explained, 'and I'm doing my thing and both of my sisters are very cool and in the know and I was at dinner with them and they were just like, *You're super ashy. You've got acne, give me your fucking credit card*, so I did and they bought me a whole bunch of super fancy French products. I have no idea what they are, but since that point I just use them every single day.'

Dudum didn't end up selling the 'super fancy French products' he claims he still can't identify unless a woman is nearby. Instead, he designed a model for subscribing to prescription medicine online (on-call doctors approve the prescriptions after a phone or email correspondence) to treat common male complaints: baldness, erectile dysfunction, and acne. What Dudum suspected was that men are ashamed to discuss these issues face-to-face but feel safe and secure using prescription drugs. Also, that while the 'who me?' detachment and self-effacement he experienced when discussing grooming and health were typical, speaking to men in an ironic bro-speak and semi-ironic baby talk might lure men toward something as embarrassing and unmanly as self-care. 'Get hard for 95% cheaper than Viagra,' reads the copy accompanying the purchase page for sildenafil – a generic form of Viagra. 'Sexy time is meant to be sexy... Ain't no one have time for bad sexy time.' This type of casual, silly, and even salty language is commonplace in ads trying to lure men; it asserts an entitled separation from the need to take matters of physical appearance and the body too seriously. When Gwyneth Paltrow sent out a newsletter in 2019 announcing that Goop would be expanding its coverage to men, she wrote: 'Click on stuff, read stuff – fuck it, go on a cleanse.' Seamus Mullen, a wellness chef who had joined her #goopfellas staff, regularly published comments like this one: 'I got to a point where my body was like Fuck you, asshole. And I had to listen.'

(When Hims begat Hers, among the first products it sold was a prescription pill often referred to as female Viagra.)

In business terms, the Hims and Hers concept is a subscription model and thus 'sticky,' meaning that once customers dip a toe in, they are stuck, credit cards and Apple Pay accounts automatically charged month after month after month after month. Whether or not the cactus remains upright, customers are unlikely to cancel their subscriptions; subscription services do remarkably well with attrition. It's the same model Goop employs with its vitamin protocols and that Amazon offers for household staples like toilet paper and dish soap. Hims competitors like Roman (same products at similar prices, businesslike photographs of its medical advisory board including the former U.S. surgeon general Dr Joycelyn Elders, and dry clinical descriptions of the available drugs) offer it, too.

BIOHACKING

BIOHACKING AS AN IDEA HAS been around since the late 1980s, but it was popularized around 2009 by a man named Dave Asprey who was, once upon a time, a three-hundred-pound computer engineer who could figure out complex coding sequences but couldn't manage his own weight until he began understanding and treating his body as a machine. When dealing with a machine, Asprey was entirely in control, and what was his body, if not a great big heaving machine of data-producing muscle, bones, and hairy, pockmarked flesh? All machine systems can be measured and improved, he reasoned. Why not this one?

If the framing here already sounds worlds away from most topics in this book, it is and it isn't. The essence of biohacking is classic wellness culture, borrowing a notion from Halbert Dunn: 'maximizing the potential of which the individual is capable.' But the prominent faces of biohacking are a data-driven, benchmark-obsessed boys' club, creating one of the biggest gender divides in wellness and departing from the ostensibly feminine, right-brain branding so prevalent elsewhere in the wellness industry.

Then again, in the age of Big Data, maybe hacking is for everyone. One biohacker, 'Quantified Bob,' explained its joys like this: 'I was always kind of obsessed with understanding what sort of knobs I could turn that adjust performance.' On his stereo, on his computer, on himself.

The nonstop, twenty-four-hour-a-day information stream provided by Dr Google and WebMD and the ClevelandClinic.com and hms.harvard.edu and the many, many websites like these, combined with the unprecedented availability of health monitoring gadgets that can be used at home, means that biohacking is an accessible 'hobby' for anyone with decent Wi-Fi. Asprey, who now runs a biohacking empire, does his own research and got his start by ordering a bunch of off-label pills from Europe. He still takes all of them, and, when we met so I could interview him about all of this, he kicked things off by disappearing beneath the table for a minute and then emerged sniffing. It was so strange! 'What did you just do?' I asked, because it seemed as if he had just done a line of cocaine in a midtown Manhattan hotel lobby shortly after 11:00 a.m.

'I just micro-dosed some nicotine,' he said, laughing. His eyes had gone a bit wild, and his fleshy pink cheeks looked somehow fleshier, definitely pinker. 'I want you to have the best possible interview.' He showed me a small, pen-like inhaler contraption manufactured by Nicorette and then acknowledged that it is neither approved nor legally available in the United States.

To understand what constitutes a biohack, start with something simple, like coffee. It's hardly news that years' worth of research shows that the caffeine in coffee has a mild stimulant effect on the nervous system, which therefore has the potential to increase productivity. With experimentation and maybe even a bit of data tracking, it's possible to figure out the exact dosage that helps you function at your highest potential. It sounds simple, but that's it: taking the information and products that are out there, gathering the data, and making it all work for you.

In talking to Dave, I realized that I'd been casually doing this already. Every morning I weigh myself on a scale that tells me not only my weight but also the percentage of me that is muscle, water, and bone. It calculates my BMI, and then it beams all that info to an app on my phone, which speaks to the other apps on my phone. My scale information talks to my Fitbit information: how much I slept, during how much of that sleep my heart rate was below resting, the number of times I wiggled and squirmed, the milliseconds between the beats of my heart, and so on. It's an astonishing amount of information to gather in the first thirty seconds of my day – unthinkable even one generation ago – and all that is accomplished using equipment with a combined cost of under $500.

Dave Asprey's big biohack is his proprietary blend of low-mold coffee (according to Asprey, so-called regular coffee 'steals your mental edge and actually makes you weak') doctored up with grass-fed butter and coconut oil. (The push for 'low-mold' coffee is a typically confusing wellness trope. The molds Asprey refers to secrete mycotoxins, which are compounds found not just in coffee but also in raisins, dark chocolate, beer, and peanut butter. The levels found in coffee are easily neutralized by a healthy liver; a study detected levels of 2–3 percent of the daily allowance for mycotoxins in about four cups of coffee. Low-mold coffee is, guess what, more expensive and shown to have little actual benefit.)

According to Asprey, his trademarked Bulletproof coffee can 'supercharge your morning,' help you lose weight, support your microbiome, and make you rich, happy, and sexually on fire. His own life is his best advertisement: he moved his family to an organic farm (where he can ensure that his food supply is truly organic) on Vancouver Island (pine trees there are known for their longevity), takes about 150 vitamins and supplements a day, bathes regularly in infrared light, hangs out in a hyperbaric chamber, and wears a rotating series of sunglasses (his own TrueDark brand) that control the types of light that make it into his brain. It's all for sale: Asprey is an evangelist for his multiple businesses. At the Bulletproof coffee shop in Santa Monica, the floor was 'electrically grounded,' the lighting is 'circadian compliant,' and the water is charcoal filtered.

Crucial to the biohacking trend is the belief in one's inner 'superhero,' an alter ego whose fundamental masculinity has been obscured by the plush conditions inherent to modern life. A lot of biohackers work intensely with their minds at their day jobs, hacking systems, designing mechanisms that have fundamentally changed almost every part of how we live. The temptation to exert the same control over one's health is extremely strong, if you are a person who likes to collect and manipulate data. If you've figured out how to store all of our music and photographs in the cloud and begun the process of replacing humans with bots to mow the lawn, vacuum the TV room, take your tolls, check you out at CVS, drive your car, and take out your appendix, how hard could controlling one lousy body be?

The superhero avatars are everywhere you look, at least in certain circles. There are the before-after pictures of Jeff Bezos and Mark Zuckerberg: Magic Mike bodies replacing poor posture and schlub (expensive personal trainers sold separately). When Jack Dorsey described his routine on a fitness podcast in March 2019, it shocked many outside the wellness and biohacking world, but few within it. Dorsey checks all the important boxes. He starts his day with an act of aggressive mindfulness: submerging his still-warm self in a freezing-cold bath – 'it just unlocks this thing in my mind and I feel like if I can will myself to do that thing that seems so small but hurts so much, I can do nearly anything' – and then he meditates. He does only seven-minute workouts; only suckers do more. He works (at his standing desk) in the glow of an infrared bulb and switches between saunas and ice baths in the evening. He's a big fan of intermittent fasting: Five days a week he eats only dinner, which he says gives him a 'very focused point of mind, and certainly the time back from breakfast and lunch allowed me to focus more on what my day is.' On the other two days, he eats nothing at all.

Dorsey is famous, so his regime is studied, but it's not only the gods of Silicon Valley who participate. There are also entrepreneurs like Serge Faguet, a thirty-eight-year-old man who lives and works in the Valley and who by 2018 had spent around $250,000 'hacking' himself. Faguet wears a pair of $6,000 hearing aids to enhance his hearing in public (there is nothing wrong with his hearing) and an Oura ring to monitor his sleep. He continuously measures his glucose levels via a subcutaneous probe that streams data to his smartphone. He injects himself with somatropin, a hormone that promotes muscle growth. He takes about sixty pills a day (an SSRI antidepressant being one of them) for a bunch of conditions he does not (yet) have. He meditates daily and follows a strict diet heavy in omega-3s. Sex is important for optimal health (*release!*), but relationships can be a drain on his performance, so Faguet has regular assignations with paid 'sugar baby models.'

Wim Hof, aka the Iceman, a bearded Dutchman who until recently held the Guinness World Record for the fastest half marathon run barefoot on ice (it was two hours, sixteen minutes, and thirty-four seconds), is another icon of male wellness. He ran this marathon above the Arctic Circle wearing only a pair of teeny-tiny shorts. Hof believes that the secret to managing disease symptoms and mastering your body has in part to do with freezing it, as you would with a lasagna you'd like to last an extra week or two. A journalist who accompanied Hof on a trip up Kilimanjaro in 2016 wrote a book about the experience called *What Doesn't Kill Us: How Freezing Water, Extreme Altitude, and Environmental Conditioning Will Renew Our Lost Evolutionary Strength*. Hof, who lives in Amsterdam, travels the world administering seminars and training sessions to audiences that are usually around 90 percent male.

This notion of heightened performance as opposed to

improved appearance is far more typical in male than in female wellness, and the men with large followings in the category typically describe themselves as superhuman robot hybrids and bots. The author Steven Kotler wrote *The Rise of Superman*, a book that describes an optimal state of consciousness that he calls 'flow' in which humans outperform their perceived abilities by getting into the 'flow' state. The book's subtitle is 'Decoding the Science of Ultimate Human Performance.'

As Maya Dusenbery put it to me, 'Men just aren't conditioned to talk about mental health issues, so it's fine to be a male athlete who is doing the stuff to enhance his performance, but that's different than doing this stuff as self-care; that seems like a more feminine vibe.' There is less discussion of spirituality in the male wellness sphere, less emphasis on nurture.

Ben Greenfield, a male wellness 'celebrity,' describes himself as a 'biohacker, human body and brain performance coach, ex-bodybuilder, Ironman triathlete, professional Spartan athlete, anti-aging consultant,' and other things, too. He takes credit 'for maximizing performance, recovery, fat loss, digestion, brain, sleep and hormone optimization for CEO's, ultra-endurance competitors, and a wide variety of professional athletes, including poker champions.' One of Greenfield's self-published books is called *The Essential Guide to Becoming Superhuman*. Greenfield opens his weekly podcast episodes by listing his credentials:

> I have a master's degree in physiology, biomechanics, and human nutrition. I've spent the past two decades competing in some of the most masochistic events on the planet from SEALFIT Kokoro, Spartan Agoge, the world's toughest mudder, the thirteen Ironman triathlons, brutal bow hunts, adventure racing, spearfishing, plant foraging, free diving, bodybuilding, and beyond. I combine this intense time in the trenches with a blend of ancestral wisdom and

BIOHACKING

modern science, search the globe for the world's top experts in performance, fat loss, recovery, gut hormones, brain, beauty, and brawn to deliver you this podcast. Everything you need to know to live an adventurous, joyful, and fulfilling life. My name is Ben Greenfield. Enjoy the ride.

Ben Greenfield sells a lot of the same products, and promises, as his female counterparts: the banishment of toxins, the balancing of hormones, the extremely optimal functioning of the body and the mind. And he is everywhere, posing waxed and topless sharing his steak recipe while standing, knife in hand, in front of a raw, fatty rack of ribs. In 2017, Greenfield underwent expensive, painful penis injections typically reserved for men with severe erectile dysfunction in an attempt to improve his orgasm. 'I wanted to go from good to great,' he said, 'and to get a bigger dick.' In the early days of COVID, Greenfield recommended a $6,000 at-home ozone generator for 'daily rectal ozone insufflation.' His endorsement? 'I'm pretty careful with what I stick up my ass.'

To the biohacked man, unwellness is an adversary. Dave Asprey wrote a blog post called 'What I Do to Protect Myself from Coronavirus, and How I Plan to Kick It if I Get It.' In it, he wrote: 'I'm sure there are people who will stand up and say, "There is no evidence that this or that works." News flash: no one knows how to cure coronavirus, so what are we going to do? We're going to be better than average.'

Biohacked men like marathons, triathlons, and *ultra*marathons. Rich Roll, who chronicles his transformation from overweight alcoholic addict to superhero in *Finding Ultra: Rejecting Middle Age, Becoming One of the World's Fittest Men, and Discovering Myself*, begins his bio with his credentials as a Stanford and Cornell graduate. It continues, 'Rich is a 50 year old accomplished vegan ultra-endurance athlete and former entertainment attorney turned full-time wellness and plant based nutrition advocate, popular public speaker, husband and father of 4 and inspiration to people worldwide as a transformative example of courageous and healthy living.' A lot of Roll's credentials have to do with the extreme races he has done: consecutive Ironman-distance triathlons under the punishing Hawaiian sun and so on.

Yet biohackers also appreciate subtlety – the smallest trigger for suboptimal performance, the untried angle of attunement. This can lead back to well-trod wellness ground. Modern Western medicine looks for big problems and then seeks to fix them, but if you go to a functional medicine doctor you will be tested for even minor food 'sensitivities,' which is a category less serious than a full-on allergy, but maybe an extra edge in your quest to be the highest-functioning you. A 'sensitivity' doesn't mean hives or anaphylaxis; it means more bloating, sadness, gas. 'Brain fog,' which is hard to pinpoint, treat, and diagnose and would likely, in earlier generations, be described as a problem of laziness or something else, has become a validated symptom.

With so much unknowable, the lure of data is intense. But the great irony is that for all these Quantified Bobs, there is as yet no long-term data. Wim Hof, running up mountains in his underpants, is hardly a reasonable control group, and the breadth of holistic medicine has yet to be harnessed in double-blind peer-reviewed fashion. So the biohackers rely on entirely anecdotal evidence, with the success of their ventures and the definition of their abs as proof that it's not all for naught.

It's not that women don't biohack. We check our steps on our phone; we monitor our scales: *I eat the pie; the number goes up. I skip the pie; down it goes again.* I've heard it called the Labracadabra effect. A joke, because there's zero magic involved in such obsessive monitoring, but it can certainly lead to any number of ta-das. And we're not immune to a little competition.

What got me to wade further into the numbers game was the dream of a good night's sleep. I don't think I am unusual in that

Biohacking

I want sleep, I need sleep, I *love* sleep. When I am awake, I often find that I miss sleep. Conveniently, sleep, which we all do and which is allegedly free, is one consistent cornerstone of pretty much every wellness regimen. It's also an area consistently described as hackable.

The bible of sleep is by Matthew Walker, a Berkeley professor of neuroscience and psychology who runs the Center for Human Sleep Science. He is the author of *Why We Sleep*, which is an extremely compelling read full of juicy and memorable facts, like the one about how car accidents caused by sleep-deprived drivers tend to be far more deadly than those caused by alcohol or drugs. And that less than six hours of sleep a night notably increases your risk of certain types of cancer. That 'our lack of sleep is a slow form of self-euthanasia,' and 'not sleeping enough, which for a portion of the population is a voluntary choice, may modify your gene transcriptome – that is, the very essence of you, or at least you as defined biologically by your DNA. Neglecting sleep could therefore represent a strange form of genetic engineering tampering with the nucleic alphabet that spells out your daily health story.'

Most people I know have experimented with sleep, during college all-nighters or red-eye flights, or new-parent marathons of pacing and feeding and the singing of songs, and the results are consistent: the quickest way to feel terrible is not to sleep. The great irony – or, in wellness business terms, opportunity – is that as we age, sleep tends to grow less reliable, less manageable. For most adults, there's no guarantee that an early bedtime will yield a delicious eight hours of rest, if the small hours will be spent calculating, worrying, regretting, wondering. For even the most exhausted, it can become more and more rare to make it to the alarm.

Sleep hygiene is not about actual cleanliness but about cleanliness of habit (except that there is a wellness pillow company called enVy that sells a $200 range of pillows that promise both neck support and 'copper ions' to combat germs and are recommended by Dave Asprey, who cites a report saying that by the end of one week, the average pillowcase harbors 3 million bacteria, which is 17,000 times more than a toilet seat).

Sleep monitors are common, relatively inexpensive, and highly addictive pieces of wearable technology that offer a continuous feed of extremely specific information.

Take the Oura ring, a sleek little device that can read like a bit of industrial-chic jewelry. The Oura ring gathers mountains of data from your finger and streams it to an app, along with pointers. Time to get up and move around. Time to power down for the day. Go to bed. NOW! I used an Oura ring for a while and then switched to a Fitbit when it included the same information as the Oura but counted my steps and my 'cardio fitness score,' too. The first thing I do every morning is retrieve my phone from a different room (wellness!), and I immediately check my sleep stats.

The frustration of the B student is intense! I've tried all the tricks: the lavender sprays, the gratitude journals, the cold showers and warm baths, and the dimming of the lights in my house at sunset so that no one can even read a book. When I remember, I wear expensive blue-light-filtering glasses (I found some more to my taste than Asprey's version; they're by a company called Felix Gray) and use an app called Oak that has a particularly soothing 'rain sounds' choice.

But and still! I just can't seem to get my sleep score up. I toss, I turn. I wake up, or I don't get enough deep sleep, or I get enough sleep, but I don't get enough REM sleep, or I fall asleep while snuggling a child or watching television and then have to get up and brush my teeth, and then the whole effort is shot before it's even 11:00 p.m. There's no quantifier for how agitation over my poor sleep score is affecting my sleep: sometimes I wake up feeling perfectly fine. I rub my eyes, I get in the shower, I turn on the kettle for tea. I feel optimistic about the day, peaceful even, but then my score scolds me. Maybe it took too long for my heart rate to settle, maybe my HRV (heart rate variability, which is the fluctuation in the intervals between adjacent heartbeats) was not ideal, and then I approach the day with more caution, a bit of dread, the expectation that I will not – could not possibly! – be at my very best. Gwyneth Paltrow's competitive streak was unleashed by Kim Kardashian's outrageously high Oura scores. 'Okay WHAT?' Paltrow wrote on her Instagram, over an image of Kardashian's sleep score of 95. 'I thought I was killing it at this @ouraring game... I guess not.' (Never one to give up, Paltrow came back on Instagram Stories with a similarly high sleep score and an 'accidental' reveal of her resting heart rate. It's 49.)

Continuous glucose monitors, devices commonly prescribed to and worn by diabetics, have become just another wearable. Though they're not available over the counter, a number of wellness start-ups have closed the black market in CGMs by offering them legally via quick 'telemedicine' appointments on their sites. The idea is that even if you don't have diabetes, a CGM can nonetheless offer a more finely tuned existence by monitoring your blood sugar levels via an app on your phone twenty-four hours a day. (One start-up's tagline: 'Ditch the scale. Grab the CGM!' Joshua Steinman, an Iraq vet and a user of Levels CGM during its beta-testing period, described his experience this way on X: 'You feel a certain way. Open up the app. Scan the sensor. Immediately start to associate a certain data point with a physical sensation.' He calls it 'the associate power of visualized data.') A Lumen device (tagline: 'Hack your metabolism'), which tells me whether my body is currently in fat or carbohydrate-burning mode, offers a similar ability for monitoring a previously unmonitorable bodily function.

My experience with both the CGM and the Lumen was, frankly, exhausting. Both devices promise a steady flow of information about what is going on within your body at any given moment. The problem of figuring out why is on the user: the best way to sleuth out the source of a feeling is to match detailed diaries about consumption, exertion, and sleep with the numbers provided by the biohacking device. It is an all-consuming effort, one that makes it difficult to spend too much time or energy doing anything else. But still, I did it. With the Lumen, I could locate no meaningful patterns. With the CGM, again, everything worked the way I might expect it to: sugar caused spikes and so on.

I know so much. And I have very little idea about what to do with any of it.

Suddenly it seemed that everyone I knew was getting a full-body scan, posing for Instagram on the edge of an MRI machine looking fresh and adorable and contented wearing identical pairs of blue-gray scrubs labeled 'Prenuvo.' A little clicking reveals that Prenuvo is an MRI start-up that offers a full-body scan to anyone willing to pay $2,500 for the privilege.

A 2019 research review concluded that 'healthcare providers should not offer whole-body MRI for preventive health screening to asymptomatic subjects outside of a research setting,' noting that such scans often produce false positive or inconclusive results that require potentially unnecessary follow-up care. Professional medical societies like the American College of Preventive Medicine, the American College of Radiology, and the USDA are not convinced of its utility or efficacy. Just try telling that to a bunch of people who just watched the world endure a pandemic that still no one seems to really understand or to those accustomed to paying for an edge.

Andrew Lacy, Prenuvo's founder, is so convincing. Why wouldn't you get a scan? But then, of course, it becomes, why wouldn't you get a scan *every day*? Oh God, what if 'it' starts growing *next week*? He is also quick with deploying historical facts, albeit not always with utmost accuracy, like that the

BIOHACKING

foundational study on mammograms was done in 1913, but it took until 1976 for them to be recommended to all American women above the age of fifty. Sixty-three years of bureaucratic hurdles and scientific debate!

How many lives might have been saved?

I had my scan in midtown Manhattan, in the shadow of Madison Square Garden, in a street-level Prenuvo center sandwiched between fast-food restaurants and happy hour commuter bars. The process was simple: I lay in a loud, clanking MRI machine for an hour (watching the David Beckham documentary on Netflix), occasionally holding my breath. I had to wait a week for my results, a week during which it was easy to say to myself, at any point, what if it's starting now? What about now? What if I had scheduled my Prenuvo a week later? The company promised peace of mind, but in my case that week was spent contemplating the worst.

My scan was mostly clean: some creaky stuff in my lower back was the most exciting finding. But still, *is it starting now, how about now?* has become a dull feed in the back of my mind, where previously, there was no such thing.

I also tried out a gym called Hackd Fitness (motto: 'Data don't lie!'), where I was asked to strip down to my underpants and stand in a three-dimensional body scan – it looked a lot like the one at the airport – that would tell me how much of me is useless wobble and how much is carrying its weight, literally. Hackd's owner preemptively softened the blow by admitting that data gathered from flawed gathering devices is inherently flawed. What was I to believe when I saw the grotesque image of myself, as if rendered in melted candle wax, every lump and bump in graphic bas-relief? The data? My lying eyes?

As much as I can't unsee that scan, in retrospect I'm grateful for the fuzziness of its technology. The plausible deniability is nice (maybe those bumps were just poor 3-D rendering?), but it's also a reminder to myself that data can take us only so far. We have become so accustomed to accessing information: My children were born twenty-one months apart, and it was amazing to me that my second pregnancy involved simple forms of testing not yet available during my first. I had it all – the old stuff, the new stuff – and it still failed to reveal what we most needed to know. We express shock when blind spots remain, but we're still only human.

IMMORTALITY

AT ONE POINT WHILE RESEARCHING this book, I traveled to a small city in the Emilia-Romagna region of Italy to attend the Global Wellness Summit. The GWS, as it's known, was cofounded in 2007 by a woman named Susie Ellis who has the pert-nosed blond looks of a 1950s surf movie heroine. 'Don't you know about Susie?' another attendee whispered one day at the conference as we listened to Ellis, so fit in a pair of trim leather trousers, introduce another speaker. I had traveled all this way to the conference, but I knew very little about its founder. The story goes like this: Ellis and her identical twin sister first appeared on the scene as aerobics teachers at the Golden Door destination spa in California during the Lycra-wrapped 1970s and 1980s. In 1995, Ellis eventually left to open and work as the director of the first-ever spa at Mar-a-Lago alongside her good friend Marla Maples (Ellis was, I was told, behind the scenes while Donald Trump gave a televised tour of the spa, urging him to endorse the body wraps). Next stop was investing in a website called Spafinder.com, where her job was exactly what it sounds like. As the industry expanded into this wild thing called wellness, Ellis expanded, too, ultimately becoming chair and CEO of the Global Wellness Institute, a nonprofit that employs researchers to document the weird world of wellness and also hosts an annual summit, which is a place where you can find the great pooh-bahs of the spa industry, but also a former surgeon general of the United States speaking about the possibility of ending disease. Like, *all preventable disease.*

The conference travels around the world (Singapore, Qatar, Palm Beach); Emilia-Romagna was chosen that year because Technogym, which is one of the world's biggest makers of treadmills and elliptical machines, has a large corporate village complete with high-ceilinged meeting spaces and showrooms there and it'd offered to host, not least because the company's founder had long worked on an initiative to transform Romagna into 'the Wellness Valley.'

In Italy, fetishism for the Italian way of life — for the natural ingredients featured in the big meals eaten with family in beautiful places — was rampant, even as it was impossible to find fresh fruits and vegetables in the gray off-season beach town near Cesena where we stayed, even as packaged gluten-free grissini adorned the tables at the summit's crowning black-tie gala event. At one point, during a pasta-making demonstration, one attendee asked a translator if dried pasta is even available in Italian supermarkets at all, or if all Italian women roll it out like this every night.

The vast range of the conference's topics seemed, like the trajectory of Ellis's career, an apt metaphor for the wellness movement itself. Panels about CBD were well attended. At lunch you could find yourself next to that former surgeon general of the United States, or next to a PR person from a global hotel chain looking to increase 'wellness offerings,' or you might find yourself next to someone who teaches at a school of cosmetology close to the Cape of Good Hope. At one point, I attended a baffling presentation on something called the Wellness Moonshot, which is an aspirational campaign to end all chronic, preventable disease in the *whole entire world*, and then the following night I went to what was billed as the world's first-ever wellness fashion show, where dozens of models in spandex and sneakers walked a long catwalk in the gardens of an elaborate seaside hotel. The GWS is a jolly, well-intentioned, and often confusing event, so it was a great representation of the wellness world at large, where the solid is so often chased by the silly, and good intentions, health, and capitalism are all rolled up into an only semi-coherent, nice-smelling ball. Sometimes I found myself looking around and thinking, *Well, here they all are, the wellness experts!* And then feeling disappointed that they look like... people. Much like the senior meditators I'd met on the final day of my meditation course, these just looked like a bunch of regular old, if carefully groomed, people; some were fat, some were thin, some with frizzy, dull hair, some with sunspots, and so on. *Where are all the Benjamin Buttons?* I wondered. Where are the *well women*? At one point I stared out a window at a group of people wearing big headphones, dancing on a patio, participants in midday silent discotheque. They looked happy enough and healthy enough, but not one of them looked as if she had found the fountain of youth. *Who knows?* I told myself as I walked into a lecture on the future of diet delivery services. *Maybe they're all 106.*

The most popular speaker of the week was Dan Buettner, the author of a series of bestselling books on longevity called *The Blue Zones*. Buettner is handsome and tan and charismatic; he wears his shirts a *little* extra unbuttoned, and he peppers his talk with irreverent jokes. He has spent the past twenty years studying Blue Zones, which is the name he gave to areas of the world where people tend to live the longest with the lowest incidence of chronic disease. Buettner has worked with a big team of demographers to identify these regions, and then to apply a microscope to the people who live in them. What do they eat? How much do they sleep? How do they get so old and stay so well? What united this disparate collection of people was the desire to juice a little extra out of life, last a little longer on earth.

The first five Blue Zones identified by Buettner were a

cluster of villages in Sardinia, the Okinawa islands in Japan, the Nicoya Peninsula in Costa Rica, the Greek island of Ikaria, and a community of Seventh-Day Adventists in San Bernardino County, California. These are places, Buettner writes, where people 'enjoy up to a 3 times better chance of reaching 100 than we do.' He told us the story of an immigrant who achieved the American dream – suburban house, car, good job – but was diagnosed with terminal lung cancer. He decided to spend the six months his American doctors told him were all he had left back home in Ikaria, where he started drinking the wine and chatting with his friends and going to church, and now that whole American cancer thing is a charming anecdote recounted by a proud centenarian.

The Blue Zone communities all sound like what the German Lebensreformers were lamenting: simple, earthbound lives, defined by community and a low-level interference from the rest of the too-modern world. (What Buettner doesn't dwell on is that these are largely homogeneous communities.) Buettner's audiences listen, eager *not* to die of cancer like that zillion-year-old Greek man, to be happy and well at a hundred and beyond by joining and implementing the rules of the 'Blue Zones Project,' whereby Buettner sells tools and plans to communities eager to become the Blue Zones of tomorrow. He also sells a Blue Zone meal plan that includes 'thousands of recipes inspired by the traditions of the world's longest lived people,' like Adventist Rice Salad and Okinawan Cream of Mushroom Soup.

Because longevity, and even immortality, are the natural end points for all of wellness. And not just living forever but living forever with a tight ass and the springy energy of freshman year, extended in perpetuity.

Many of the biohackers are aspiring immortals. Dave Asprey says he'll live to 180 ('at least, I don't want to limit myself,' he told me) and that if he and his physician wife decide to have another round of kids in their eighties, well, why not? Who would carry them? I ask.

'Well, she would,' he says, 'or I would if I want to.' So we await the possibility of low-mold-coffee Dave becoming the world's first eighty-five-year-old pregnant man.

The tech supermen are also on board for defeating death, of course. Sergey Brin, the Google cofounder whose ex-wife cofounded the genetic testing company 23andMe, learned thereby that he had a genetic predisposition to developing Parkinson's disease. Five years later, Google invested $1 billion to launch a secretive company called Calico – short for California Life Company – which focuses on longevity research. Jeff Bezos is one of the investors in Unity, a longevity biotech company led by a middle-aged man named Ned David whose youthful looks perhaps convince investors of the efficacy of his approach. One start-up founder told *The New Yorker*'s Tad Friend, 'The proposition that we can live forever is obvious. It doesn't violate the laws of physics, so we will achieve it.'

There's a doctor who runs a hedge fund in California named Joon Yun whose interest is in preserving not only the length but also the quality of life. Both, he believes, are infinitely possible in a healthy person – 'There is no difference between longevity and wellness,' he told me – and then he offers a, to me, perfect definition of wellness: it is nothing. It's just a feeling of peace so complete that the feeling itself disappears. Wellness is the absence of irritation, a feeling of lightness and ease, both mental and physical. It is sleep that comes when the lids first close and lasts – deep and black – exactly as long as you need. It is waking up sparkling, ready, refreshed. It is a body free from aches, pains, scars. If you are truly well and you trip and fall, you'll soon be up again, and any pain, discomfort, or embarrassment will recede swiftly and completely. A perpetual life machine.

Recently, tabloids, but also the mainstream press, have enjoyed telling the story of a California man named Bryan

Johnson who sold an online payment company he'd founded and upon netting $300 million decided to spend some large portion of that on… his physical self. Not only does he want to live forever, but he wants to reverse his biological age. In 2023 he was forty-five in chronological years but spending all day every day attempting to nudge any measurable quantifiers of his health to match those of a typical teenage boy. He was also spending around $2 million a year on the effort and taking 111 pills a day. It 'has produced near perfect health for me,' he says proudly. He'd injected himself with his teenage son's blood plasma, but stopped after detecting no measurable benefit.

Back at the Global Wellness Summit, Dan Buettner was ready to reveal the secrets of his long-lived Blue Zones. But first he asked the audience to respond to eight questions:

Raise your hand if…
You sleep at least seven hours a night.
You move for at least thirty minutes a day.
You eat three honest servings of vegetables every day.
You have not had unprotected sex with a stranger ('I want to party with you guys tonight!').
You belong to a faith, and keep your hand up if you show up at least four times a month.
You have at least three friends who you can have a meaningful conversation with, call on a bad day and they'd care, and you actually like.
You have not smoked tobacco in the last five years.
You have the desire and the physical capacity to live to the age of ninety.

The closer you got to eight 'yes' answers, the more well you are, Buettner explained. There are no potions or tablets or saunas or steams that matter, and 'no matter where you go in the world and you see long-living people, it's not because they tried. They never said at age fifty, "I'm going to get on that longevity diet and live another fifty years,"' he said. 'They didn't join the wellness program at work; they didn't call up a 1-800 number and start ordering supplements. The big epiphany here is that longevity is not something that is successfully pursued.'

I watched the shoulders of a woman I'd just seen on a panel discussion on corporate wellness slump. When I'd wandered into the room where she'd been speaking an hour earlier, she was imploring her audience, 'But how do you get people to *come*?' I, great ignorer of HR emails, slinked out the back and went to another talk about CBD. And now here we all were, the surgeon general and the facialist and the architect interested in the healing powers of light, and none of it mattered at all. Living a long, healthy, beautiful life, we were being told, is not something that can be taught or bought or even meaningfully pursued. Everyone liked Dan Buettner, but it was hard not to feel a little silly if you'd just spent a few hundred bucks on probiotics and adaptogens and then watched a slideshow starring a 105-year-old Adventist who would never do that and who still bikes to her volunteer job… at an old-folks home (ba-dum-*bum*).

Buettner had entered his project with mixed expectations, keeping in mind a report issued by fifty-one of the world's top longevity experts in 2002 that read: 'Our language on this matter must be unambiguous. There are no lifestyle changes, surgical procedures, vitamins, antioxidants, hormones, or techniques of genetic engineering available today that have been demonstrated to influence the processes of aging.'

Even with this 'there are no secrets' answer, he would still go on to write four bestselling books, still travel the world delivering this 'raise your hand' speech (sometimes as a TED talk) to eager people who sit, with pens poised above notebooks, smiling at the story of an elderly cancer-beating Greek.

How To Be Well

I took a quiz on the Blue Zones website that told me that, given my current habits, I'm on track to live to 91.8, but that I could, using Blue Zone methodology, make it to 97.4. The free advice was to sleep more, drink red wine, be friendlier ('It may not surprise you to hear that a new friend can help you live longer, but did you know friends can be worth $134,000 of happiness?'), find faith (all but 5 of the 263 centenarians studied by the Blue Zone team described regular, faith-based practices), and improve my attitude. That last bit was generated when I'd admitted to feeling stress, anger, and sadness in the previous thirty days on the questionnaire. Some of the advice was accompanied by articles like '5 Rules for Building True Friendships' that I could read for free. If I wanted other advice, like the Blue Zones guide to better sleep, I'd have to pay, and I didn't want to pay. Also, my Modern Age clinic evaluation had told me — even before I subjected myself to an hour-long vitamin drip — that my physical age is three years younger than my chronological age. So maybe this means I'm on track to live to 94.8, anyway, and certainly that's plenty?

The biohacked body and mind are not unlike cryptocurrency: a great big bet on an unknowable future. We see biohacked people with their shirts off, with abs ripped well past the point where one might reasonably expect such a thing, and determine that biohacking is working for them. When meditators swear by their meditations, attributing Super Bowl wins and mega-celebrity and extreme corporate and business successes to the practice, such a practice begins to seem unassailable. Its benefit is suggested in each of my meditation instructor's tinkly giggles, in the ever-friendly squinting of his nicely crinkled eyes.

But there is not yet evidence on the big stuff, on whether and to what extent it is possible to improve upon the general level of health that affluence in America can afford. We know that some level of privilege, access, and vigilance can prevent the worst outcomes, but we don't yet understand what these 'better' outcomes might look like. When I open my eyes at the end of a meditation, I have not transcended. I am still in the small purple chair in my room, the facts of my life unmoved by my effort. My fellow meditators seem much the same: regular people just trying to make it through another day.

Most of the women I know do not actually want to live forever. Not on this earth, not in the ether or the cloud or anywhere else. What women tend to want, I've found, is to live for a good long while in a suspended state. Immortality just seems... exhausting.

The grand finale of my meditation class was a big group session with previous graduates. Michael Miller, our teacher, threw open the doors to the gallery, and the meditators flooded in. They didn't look particularly optimized, not like corporate raiders, or like celestial beings, or like anything really but a pretty random cross section of the types of people one sees around New York in the hours when work wraps up: well-intentioned working people, not hippies, just people. Tired from the struggle, the schlep. As everyone sat there, eyes closed, foreheads gently furrowing, it felt hard to be cynical or skeptical about a roomful of people so hungry for a moment of stillness and peace. Are we really all trying to take over the world? Or has the endlessly aggressive selling of it all obscured the most basic and simple fact that we are all, ultimately, just looking for a tiny bit of peace.

CONCLUSION

Throughout the course of writing this book, I have been asked the same question over and over: What *actually* works? What is the one thing I should be doing to become this magic woman? Is there a secret something that's worth the trouble? I would love to be able to whisper, conspiratorially, *It's ashwagandha!!* And then go home and draw up plans for a lucrative ashwagandha concern. Or come up with a nine-point checklist, easily managed on a paid subscription app. *Lock yourself in this closet three times a week!* I'd say at every cocktail party. *Eat only this terrible pile of nuts! You will look beautiful, you will feel safe, you will live forever and beyond, you will suffer no more, nor will any of the people you love! You will be the well-est of women.* I can see the disappointment when I answer, 'Oh, you know, the usual…' The longing for a magic fountain or bullet or secret is strong.

I came across the words of a Boston academic named Carol-Ann Farkas, who in a paper examining the advice given in health and wellness magazines wrote: 'Though our vigilant pursuit of health information may fuel an obsessive-compulsive mix of hypochondria and consumerism, it may also result in our acquiring a great deal of expertise about ourselves; sooner or later we will learn something and acquire power from that knowledge.'

Have I learned anything from studying this seductive blend of hypochondria and buying stuff?

Conclusion

Here's what I have learned: as fancy as it might seem to say, 'I avoid hybridized wheat,' the knowledge of the lay hobbyist is still minute considering the vast complexity of the human body, chemical science, and the constantly evolving ways in which our food and products are made and consumed. It's tempting to take the kernels of truth gleaned from 'studies' summarized on beautifully designed websites and run with them, to fill in the gaps in our knowledge with what can seem logical, and compelling, narrative.

There is no question that some aspects of the wellness movement have the benefit of enabling new groups of people to be legitimized and heard in their complaints. Also, there are the seeds of new options for treatment that consider the many mysteries and vicissitudes of the human condition. In this arena, one hopes it is only a start, but also that the progress made is not derailed by profit motives and greed. I am constantly alarmed by how many of the well-founded fears associated with traditional medicine are being replicated in wellness alternatives. Do we not worry that products labeled 'organic' might also build up in our organs and blood? That they might contain dangerous and untested elements, too? It's true that we just don't know what the long-term effects of many common consumer chemicals might be on our health, but this is also true of the vitamins and dusts we are sold as a way to cope, and it is also more true of the many exposures we do not control than it is of the ones that we do. Medicine has surely been corrupted by the pressures of Big Pharma, but many alternative and functional doctors push proprietary, for-profit lines of supplements. And while the body and the mind are obviously linked (imagine a world in which they were not! How would that work?), I refuse the patient blaming that comes with too much emphasis on the power of positive thought.

An overwhelming fixation on how bodies look has marked my life and the lives of too many women I know, and the enduring lesson I've taken away from all this time in the magical world of well has to do with how easily disordered behaviors slip from health practice to unhealthy practice. When we intermittently fast, commit to invasive purging, eliminate entire categories of food, play any version of these all-too-familiar games of chicken with our natural appetites, hungers, and satiety, I can confidently say that we are replicating what are elsewhere diagnosed as unhealthy and disordered relationships to eating and food. So much of what is pushed on us in the name of being healthy stinks of what we decry as its opposite. Women are forever being criticized and sold solutions, and this time is less different than we think.

This book — as well as my desire to understand the wellness movement in general — is really a love letter to my daughters. I want more for them than the endless chasing, chasing, chasing of self-improvement that can easily define modern American womanhood. I want their health to be valued and prioritized, and I do not want endemic striving to dominate their lives.

During my research I read a fascinating book called *The Body Project*, for which the historian Joan Jacobs Brumberg read hundreds of diary entries by adolescent girls from over the past century. What is striking is the consistent yearning to better oneself that changes not in mission but in form. In 1892, a typical diary entry read, 'Resolved, not to talk about myself or feelings. To think before speaking. To work seriously. To be self-restrained in conversation and action. Not to let my thoughts wander. To be dignified. Interest myself more in others.' An entry dated 1982 sounds more familiar: 'I will try to make myself better in any way I possibly can with the help of my budget and babysitting money. I will lose weight, get new lenses, already got new haircut, good makeup, new clothes and accessories.' Brumberg's book was published in 1997, and one can only imagine journals by teenage girls now who disavow gluten and milk, make promises about Transcendental Meditation practices, and promise to evict something 'toxic' and replace it with something 'clean.' They diagnose themselves and their friends freely, announce when they are 'disassociating,' speculate about who is on which spectrum and why, allow these traits and conditions to define themselves and their identities. These previously private stirrings and strivings might well take place in the public forums of social media, where other girls might comment on whether any of it is working at all. On a recent trip to Barnes & Noble to buy a plain, lined journal, I had a hard time finding one that was not full of wellness prompts: ordered spaces designated for the setting of intentions and expressions of gratitude, a sleeve of stickers to denote the successful honoring of one's body and mind, the small victories of self-control that deny easy, cheap pleasures in favor of a larger goal.

I think we owe it to our daughters to draw firmer boundaries around what is expected of them as women, which might work if we are better about treating their legitimate concerns legitimately. Ideally, we would be capable of holding opposing ideas as simultaneously true: managing the wellness industry's murky contradictions, extracting what serves us, discarding what does not. 'Wellness' is not going anywhere; it will be our project to make sure it doesn't eat us alive.

Here's what I know to be true: Drink enough water. Sleep as much as you can. Eat big leafy greens instead of things you can't pronounce. Move your body around as much as you can, preferably in nature, and hope that you find some sort of faith in a force bigger than yourself. Spend time with friends, love your family, don't work all the time. Look for the best medical care you can manage and a doctor who listens when you talk. Also, don't monitor yourself too obsessively, or you're liable to go nuts.

Mostly: remember that things that are for sale are not always what they seem.

How To Be Well

What I hope for my daughters, for all of us, is that we find a way to be happy, content, healthy, and well; that our society will do a better job of supporting this mission; and that we will not be asked to spend so much of our time and money addressing the many, many ways in which we will all, inevitably, fall short all the time, always.

And yet.

It's probably too late for me. I remain hopeful. I don't stop wondering if there is some secret sauce out there, some fountain of something that's better than this. The constant barrage of wellness out there in the world I inhabit makes it hard not to: if I get an email with the heading 'Top Summer Beauty and Wellness Tips!' from the makeup artist turned wellness guru Bobbi Brown, I will click it open and, down deep inside, I will wonder if this is the one that will unlock a brand-new truth. And when it doesn't, when the tips are all 'Stop worrying about mascara smears and try eyelash extensions!' I will still click on the next email from Bobbi Brown and curiously scan the suggestions, thinking, *Well, you never know!*

Even though I do know.

With managed expectations there's plenty of fun to be had in the wild world of wellness, just as there is with lipstick or a new pair of shoes. I do not expect or require anyone to give any of it up, particularly if – to borrow Marie Kondo's expression – it sparks joy.

Don't stop speaking up about discomfort, don't stop looking for a better alternative, don't stop advocating for yourself, but remain conscious of the limits. No matter how many wacky wellness remedies I try, plenty of new little lines show up around my eyes, above my lips. The spots on my hands multiply and spread. My right shoulder still locks up sometimes, though I guess there's no way to know if, without all those Pilates sessions, foam rolling, the cold cryo, the scary infrared Freddy

Conclusion

Krueger LED-light mask, the wrinkles would have had greater depth, my shoulder would hurt even more.

I didn't fly out of Diane's office after that horrible colonic. It was more of a shuffle, really, and I spent a lot of time over the next few days wondering when the gas pains would stop and worrying about the same old crap I'd been worrying about when I went in. The world outside my house didn't get any better; in a number of hideous and obvious ways, it got even worse.

I decided, in the end, to skip the psychedelics: my limited experience with psychedelic drugs did not suggest to me that I would travel, in that midtown high-rise, to any important place. Quite the opposite. I am committed instead to doing the work I need to do on myself while I am awake.

Also, I don't want to wake up to those nipple-tweaking fuckbots.

When I engage in a little recreational wellness, I enter into the same kind of semi-complicity as the people who hire psychics and mediums to manage their grief: what I want when I spend an afternoon reading about the disappointing reality of collagen supplements (they do nothing) is to feel comforted about my impending decline, to feel that I at least put up a fight against what the poet Philip Larkin calls 'the only end of age.'

I've done cryo and infrared and meditation and juice fasts and elimination diets, and I've monitored my heartbeat, my muscle mass, my sleep cycles, and the milliseconds between the beats of my heart. I've attempted to 'hack my metabolism' using a little Breathalyzer that came in a box, and I wore a continuous glucose monitor just to see what it would say. I'm an expert in all the varieties of still-available ancient grains.

Some of what I've learned has only made me more neurotic: I've worried so much about the importance of sleep that when I do wake up at 4:00 a.m. worrying that something terrible could befall my children, my husband, my parents, my friends, I worry about whether I'm jeopardizing my own health by not sleeping in pure Huffington-ian soundness, so when I inevitably fall apart, who will take care of my children, my husband, my parents, my friends?

In the 'wellll, what if' category I have switched out some of my beauty products – deodorant, moisturizer, soap – for 'clean' versions. I can't really defend the choice. After all this research I don't fundamentally believe that the levels of toxic exposures in most common household products are dangerous, but I also can't get past the gnawing *what if, what if.* The vast majority of our 'toxic' exposures occur outside the controllable confines of my bathroom – in the air, the water, the earth itself – but knowing that, I find some comfort in being in charge of even a minuscule amount. After all, as Paracelsus first pointed out, the problem lies in the dose, so why not manage whatever teeny portion I can? I don't actually think that recycling my bottles and cans will put even the smallest of dents in climate change, but at least I'm giving it a go. My 'safe' products are all exponentially more expensive than my old ones: my old drugstore deodorant cost $3.79 a stick, and my new Corpus brand costs $22, which strikes me as offensive even if it does smell of bergamot, pink lemons, orange blossom, and cardamom. I can afford to indulge my doubt, just as I can afford to have my nails done in a salon where I am exposed to far lower amounts of phthalates than the women who work there.

Am I a well woman? The embarrassing truth is this: What is most relevant to my health is my socioeconomic status. I buy high-quality food, and my work accommodates rest. The doctors I see are uniformly great. I pay out of pocket to see my GP once a year, and she spends an hour asking me about everything, whether I'm exercising, but also the health of my marriage, kids, and parents. She listens carefully to the answers. If she recommends any follow-ups, I have the time and means

CONCLUSION

to get there. I live in a neighborhood with low rates of asthma, obesity, diabetes.

What no one wants to say is this: what you really need is to be lucky, and what is often meant by 'lucky' is rich.

None of this is fair, and, even when the odds are in your favor, there are no guarantees. My favorite wellness routine is a 4, 7, 8 breathing technique that I learned from a childhood friend who used it herself during the long illness suffered by her deeply loved husband, who died of cancer at thirty-eight when their twin sons were six months old.

In for 4, hold for 7, release for 8. There are technical reasons why it works: stress is all sympathetic nervous system; slow breathing stimulates the parasympathetic nerves, calming it all down. It's simple, logical, direct. For me, it works.

I'm pretty sure I don't want to live forever, or even how much so-called extra time I want. Will I be tired, like the fabulous family member who looks like Diane Keaton and once shocked a young stranger by saying, 'Oh, I'm so glad my turn is almost up and all of this' – she meant the fucked-up world – 'won't be my problem anymore!' Or will I be desperate for any scrap of time with my husband, my daughters, their daughters and sons, and the daughters and sons that might come after that? How important are some extra number of swims in (or even just looks at) the sea, bowls of tomato pasta, my husband's jokes, the warmth of dappled sunlight on random unremarkable afternoons? Of course I could step off a curb at the wrong moment this day or the next. I have survived the difficulties and the grief I have been dealt, but who knows what comes next? No matter how well I am, it's still coming. Climate change and viruses and wars and smaller, more personal horrors don't care that I switched out my deodorant, used mineral sunscreen, ate my body weight in leafy greens, dutifully dropped vitamin D supplements each cloudy morning onto my waiting, believing tongue.

But at least, I can tell myself when they do, *at least I tried.*

ACKNOWLEDGMENTS

This book began as a story at my longtime home, *New York* magazine, several lifetimes ago. It was brought to life with the help of great friends and collaborators David Wallace-Wells, Jody Quon, Adam Moss, and of course Jared Hohlt. Jared has been crucial at every step, from the moment I first had this idea until, probably, whatever it is I'm doing right this very minute. He is the best editor, adviser, friend, and support any sane person has the right to expect in this life, or the next.

Enormous thanks to my agent, David Kuhn, who helped me shape this idea into book form and then to sell it, enlisting the excellent Nate Muscato and the rest of the responsive and organized staff at Aevitas.

At Knopf, Lexy Bloom understood right away that wellness is far too complex a topic to be something that we are for or against, that a one-note endorsement or takedown simply would not do. I am grateful for her commitment, loyalty, and understanding through the long road we have been down together with this project. Also at Knopf, thanks to Isa Connolly, Morgan Hamilton, Nora Reichard, Kelly Shi, Erinn Hartman, Samantha Bryant, and Laura Keefe.

Meghan Houser lent a fresh and magical editorial eye when mine could no longer see, and Sameen Gauhar lent another clear perspective, as well as a detailed and thorough checking of facts.

I am grateful to the people who allowed me to interview

ACKNOWLEDGMENTS

them about their lives and their livelihoods, about their own struggles with being well enough. The interviews often detoured into personal territory, and I am grateful for the time and the trust of the many individuals I have spoken with during my research, those whose stories made it in, and those whose didn't but certainly influenced my thinking.

I also owe thanks to the practitioners who keep me up and running and feeling mostly well-ish in body and in mind: Drs. Holly Andersen and Chris Creatura, my therapist M. Kim Sarasohn, the stellar roster of classical Pilates instructors at Real Pilates in New York and Exhale in London, Rachel Warren at Forward_Space, Laurie and Lamar at Soul-Cycle, freelance Pilates wizard Laura Gunder, and Saki Kim, who not only gives the best massages, but follows them up with a homemade cookie every single time.

There are many Blue Zone categories where I fall down completely (faith, for example, will be adding zero days to this life), but when it comes to friends and family, I am lucky to knock it out of the park. Thank you to Jim and Dale Larocca, my endlessly loving and generous parents, and to my brothers, Josh and Mike, for stacking the deck for me from the start, and now to Yulun Yang and Nina Freudenberger, and to Claire and Jack and Wolfie and Jules.

My mother-in-law, Mary Kay Wilmers, and I have yet to open the London Review of Frocks, but I like to think that it's still coming and that we will offer superior services for body dysmorphics and lovers of cashmere shawls. Until we realize our shared dream, she is a constant source of love and advice, and wisdom and jokes, and to her I am grateful for so much. Sam Frears consistently inspires and redraws the boundaries of what it means to be well with his bottomless ability to find joy in life. Thank you of course, as well, to Stephen Frears, Lola Frears, Frankie Frears, and Annie Rothenstein (the one who looks like Annie Hall).

How To Be Well

My friends in New York and in London have really had to put up with an awful lot out of me: so many wellness laments! They have been very nice about the whole thing. In New York, thank God for Carolyn Glass, Jenny Comita, Sabina Schlumberger, Risa Scobie, Bonnie Morrison, Susan Burden, Natasha Jakubowski, Alexis Agathocleous, Jess Leader, Richard Fine, Jacob Weisberg, Deborah Needleman, Annie Dorsen, and again (he deserves it) for Jared Hohlt. Amanda McGovern and Sarah Min both helped me celebrate important milestones. Claudia Zelevansky deserves a medal. I can't imagine life without Ian Jackman and Kara Welsh!

Tamari Japaridze makes everything possible, as do the many wonderful women who have helped care for and serve as role models for our girls while Will and I work.

In London, Andrew O'Hagan was the best officemate (we know what we are) and early reader. Gaby Wood talked me through some of this project's stickier moments, as did Miranda Carter and John Lanchester. (There were enough sticky moments, alas, to go around.) Inigo Thomas has so often looked after me, after us all. Thank you to Seamus MacGibbon for asking if I like conversation, and to Rita Konig for so much happiness and laughing, for all the Blue Zone years she has added to my life for sure! The staff at the Trevor-Roberts School in Belsize Park kept me sane when they stayed open in the fall of 2020. I could weep with gratitude just thinking about it now.

Oceans of gratitude to Duncan Wilkins, Sophia Langmead, Annabel Moorsom, Georgie Neve, Charlie, Oscar, Wayne, Cudjoe, Dickie, Julian, and the Squad.

The great heartbreak in writing these thanks is that three of the opinions I most value would have come from three people who are no longer here. Olivia Barker, Michael Friedman, and John Homans all influenced me in deep and important ways, and I think about each of them all of the time, always.

Acknowledgments

Oona and Ruby, writing in the conclusion that this book is a love letter to the two of you isn't even the half of it. There is nothing better in the entire world (galaxy, universe, etc.) than being your mother, and, to the extent that I am good at all, it is because I know the two of you.

And to Will, for more time with you, I would do all the creepy wellness things in the world. Did I get what I wanted?

I did.

NOTES

INTRODUCTION

11 **Wellness is currently a $5.6 trillion industry:** Sarah Rappaport, 'The Global Wellness Industry Is Now Worth $5.6 Trillion,' *Bloomberg News*, Nov. 9, 2023.

11 **$29 billion across 730 deals:** 'Still Feeling Good: The U.S. Wellness Market Continues to Boom,' McKinsey & Company, Sept. 19, 2022.

14 **'I usually wake up at 6:30am':** Victoria Dawson Hoff, 'How Hollywood's Favorite Juice Bar Owner Eats Every Day,' *Elle*, May 29, 2015.

15 **The party girl known for her leather:** Louise Rafkin, 'Living with Lyme Disease, Stronger with Love,' *New York Times*, May 24, 2019.

16 **Goop's $250 million piece of the market:** Taffy Brodesser-Akner, 'How Goop's Haters Made Gwyneth Paltrow's Company Worth $250 Million,' *New York Times*, July 25, 2018.

PART I : CURE

27 **The average ER in America:** Nicos Savva and Tolga Tezcan, 'To Reduce Emergency Wait Room Times, Tie Them to Payments,' *Harvard Business Review*, Feb. 6, 2019, hbr.org.

29 **Flexner visited all 150 of the medical schools:** Abraham

Notes

Flexner, *Medical Education in the United States and Canada* (New York: Carnegie Foundation for the Advancement of Teaching, 1910).

30 **A lot of the research and testing:** Maya Dusenbery, *Doing Harm: The Truth About How Bad Medicine and Lazy Science Leave Women Dismissed, Misdiagnosed, and Sick* (New York: HarperCollins, 2017), 25.

30 **'Somehow, I find it hard to believe':** Dusenbery, *Doing Harm*, 25.

31 **In 1910, only 6 percent of doctors:** Anne Walling, Kari Nilsen, and Kimberly J. Templeton, 'The Only Woman in the Room: Oral Histories of Senior Women Physicians in a Midwestern City,' *Women's Health Reports* 1, no. 1 (2020): 279–86.

31 **by 1976 the proportion of women in medical school:** Keith Chen and Judith Chevalier, 'Is Medical School a Worthwhile Investment for Women?,' *Atlantic*, July 23, 2012.

31 **'One of the bitterest aspects':** Meghan O'Rourke, *The Invisible Kingdom: Reimagining Chronic Illness* (New York: Riverhead Books, 2022), 269.

MEDICINE AND ITS ALTERNATIVES

36 **'an integrated method of functioning':** Halbert L. Dunn, *High-Level Wellness* (Arlington, Va.: R. W. Beatty, 1961), 4–5.

37 **'state of being well':** Halbert L. Dunn, 'High-Level Wellness for Man and Society,' *American Journal of Public Health* 49 (June 1959): 786–92.

37 **'Halbert Dunn [Hal] profoundly':** https://abbottsolutionsinc.com/pdf/Travis_HLDunn_Award_Handout.pdf.

38 **'establishment view of the drug':** Andrew Weil, *The Natural Mind: An Investigation of Drugs and the Higher*

Consciousness (Boston: Houghton Mifflin Harcourt, 1998), x.

38 'exactly analogous to religious fundamentalism': 'The Believers,' *Economist*, April 14, 2012.

HOLISTIC, FUNCTIONAL, PROFITABLE

45 'I was startled by the profound discomfort': O'Rourke, *Invisible Kingdom*, 60.

46 'Upon entry, Parsley Health's light-filled': Lauren Valenti, 'Inside the New York Wellness Space That Could Be the Future of Primary Care,' *Vogue*, Jan. 30, 2019.

46 'We paid close attention to the color palette': Kara Ladd, 'This Modern Healthcare Startup Is Using Design to Heal,' *Architectural Digest,* Nov. 14, 2019.

48 **The tenets, as defined by:** William Browning, Catherine Ryan, and Joseph Clancy, *14 Patterns of Biophilic Design: Improving Health and Well-Being in the Built Environment* (New York: Terrapin Bright Green, 2014), www.terrapinbrightgreen.com.

48 **A 2016 Pew Research survey found:** Aaron Smith and Monica Anderson, 'Online Shopping and E-commerce,' Pew Research Center, Dec. 2016, www.pewinternet.org.

48 **a 2022 Raydiant study:** 'State of Consumer Behavior 2022,' Raydiant, March 2022, www.raydiant.com.

53 **'It was important to Tia':** Anne DiNardo, 'Refreshing Women's Health by Design,' *Healthcare Design*, June 27, 2022, healthcaredesignmagazine.com.

55 **'The thoughtfulness that goes into curating':** Rebecca Suhrawardi, 'As Some States Brace for Next Lockdown, the Fashion and Celebrity Set Embrace Luxury Healthcare,' *Forbes*, Dec. 1, 2020.

KOOKS

58 **'This was part of an American':** Michael Hobbes and Aubrey Gordon, 'Paul Bragg and the Rise of Apple Cider Vinegar,' *Maintenance Phase*, Oct. 11, 2022, www.maintenancephase.com.

60 **'It's one of the core beliefs':** Eva Wiseman, 'Jennifer Gunter: Women Are Being Told Lies About Their Bodies,' *Guardian*, Sept. 8, 2019.

60 **'Dear God, no':** Jen Gunter, *The Vagina Bible: The Vulva and the Vagina – Separating Myth from the Medicine* (New York: Citadel Press, 2019), 386.

60 **'The fact that individuals':** Timothy Caulfield, *Is Gwyneth Paltrow Wrong About Everything? How the Famous Sell Us Elixirs of Health, Beauty, and Happiness* (Boston: Beacon Press, 2015), 66.

63 **'The time has come for this genre':** Bill Adler, *The Uncommon Wisdom of Oprah Winfrey: A Portrait in Her Own Words* (New York: Carol, 1996), 76.

64 **In 2012, Oprah traveled to Brazil:** Oprah Winfrey, 'Oprah's Visit to John of God: You Are Exactly Where You Need to Be,' Oprah.com, March 17, 2013.

66 **so it's not entirely surprising:** Christina Korownyk et al., 'Televised Medical Talk Shows – What They Recommend and the Evidence to Support Their Recommendations: A Prospective Observational Study,' *British Medical Journal*, Dec. 2014, 349.

66 **'Dr. Oz has repeatedly shown disdain':** Julia Belluz, 'A Group of Doctors Just Asked Columbia to Reconsider Dr Oz's Faculty Appointment,' *Vox*, April 16, 2015.

67 **'I've been looking for a menopause company!':** Amy Larocca, 'Welcome to the Menopause Gold Rush,' *New York Times*, Dec. 20, 2022.

67 **Medical practitioners received a shockingly small amount:** Johns Hopkins University School of Medicine,

'What Do Ob/Gyns in Training Learn About Menopause? Not Nearly Enough, New Study Suggests,' news release, May 1, 2013.

68 **Usage of HRT immediately dropped:** Susan Dominus, 'Women Have Been Misled About Menopause,' *New York Times Magazine*, Feb. 1, 2023.

CHRONIC ILLNESS

74 **'social media's latest conqueror':** Blake Montgomery, 'Being Sick Made Them Famous – and a Target of Trolls,' *Daily Beast*, Feb. 18, 2020.

74 **'The one thing I do know':** Porochista Khakpour, *Sick: A Memoir* (New York: HarperCollins, 2018), 36.

74 **'It is no coincidence then that':** Khakpour, *Sick*, 177.

75 **'One of the punitive fantasies':** O'Rourke, *Invisible Kingdom*, 103.

75 **'the climate change of the human body':** Sarah Ramey, *The Lady's Handbook for Her Mysterious Illness: A Memoir* (New York: Knopf, 2021), 321.

76 **'It's not that women come in':** Mary Elizabeth Williams, 'Mystery Illnesses Are on the Rise with Women, Whom Doctors Are Dismissing as "Nervous Nellies,"' *Salon*, April 7, 2020.

SELF-CARE

78 **'What's the most important lesson':** Tara Parker-Pope, 'Why Self-Care Isn't Selfish,' *New York Times*, Jan. 6, 2021.

79 **93 percent of ob-gyns were men:** Soumya Karlamangla, 'Male Doctors Are Disappearing from Gynecology. Not Everybody Is Thrilled About It,' *Los Angeles Times*, March 7, 2018.

80 **82 percent of ob-gyns placed:** Alex Olgin, 'Male OB-GYNs Are Rare, but Is That a Problem?,' *Morning Edition*, NPR, April 12, 2018.

Notes

80 **'A person's health is their most valuable'**: Alondra Nelson, *Body and Soul: The Black Panther Party and the Fight Against Medical Discrimination* (Minneapolis: University of Minnesota Press, 2011), 77.

82 **'I respect the time I spend'**: Audre Lorde, *A Burst of Light, and Other Essays* (Mineola, N.Y.: Ixia Press, 2017), 128.

82 **'Sometimes I feel like I am living'**: Lorde, *A Burst of Light*, 130.

84 **'The greater one's income'**: Steven H. Woolf et al., 'How Are Income and Wealth Linked to Health and Longevity?,' Urban Institute and Virginia Commonwealth University, April 2015.

84 **death rate for Black Americans**: Latoya Hill, Samantha Artiga, and Nambi Ndugga, 'COVID-19 Cases, Deaths, and Vaccinations by Race/Ethnicity as of Winter 2022,' Kaiser Family Foundation, March 7, 2023.

84 **Black women are three times**: Donna L. Hoyert, 'Maternal Mortality Rates in the United States, 2021,' Centers for Disease Control and Prevention, www.cdc.gov.

84 **'treating myself to a massage'**: Ivanka Trump, *Women Who Work: Rewriting the Rules for Success* (New York: Portfolio, 2017), 146.

PART II: GLOW

92 **'I think that shopping at CAP'**: 'CAP Beauty on the Profound Act of Self-Care,' Feb. 28, 2018, www.jennikayne.com.

92 **Clairol ran an ad for hair dye**: Rose Weitz, *Rapunzel's Daughters: What Women's Hair Tells Us About Women's Lives* (New York: Farrar, Straus & Giroux, 2004), 192.

92 **Today, the number of American women**: Marianna Cerini, 'From Rainbow to Gray: The Evolution of Hair Dye,' CNN, March 25, 2020, www.cnn.com.

92 **'Edna's case was really a pathetic one':** Barbara Lippert, 'Listerine and the Halitosis Hallelujah,' *Ad Age*, Sept. 28, 2017.

BODY POSITIVE?

96 **'Do you know how much':** Lauren Collins, 'Pixel Perfect,' *New Yorker*, May 12, 2008.

96 **the company was in a colossal rut:** Jess Miller, 'Weight Watchers Isn't Fooling Anyone,' *Slate*, March 8, 2021, www.slate.com.

100 **the venom of the Gila monster:** Rolfe Winkler and Ben Cohen, 'Monster Diet Drugs Like Ozempic Started with Actual Monsters,' *Wall Street Journal*, June 23, 2023.

100 **Novo Nordisk, a Danish pharmaceutical company:** Dhruv Khullar, 'The Year of Ozempic,' *New Yorker*, Dec. 14, 2023.

101 **'The vast majority of fat people':** Michael Hobbes and Aubrey Gordon, 'Ozempic,' *Maintenance Phase*, Oct. 10, 2023, www.maintenancephase.com.

SEX POSITIVE

105 **'I never claimed to have evidence':** Robinson Meyer and Ashley Fetters, 'Victorian-Era Orgasms and the Crisis of Peer Review,' *Atlantic*, Sept. 6, 2018.

105 **'We spent serious time on the aesthetic':** Jennifer Berry, 'Goop's First-Ever Vibrator Is Here – and She's a Beauty,' *Fashion*, Feb. 14, 2021.

CLEAN BEAUTY

108 **'I thought I was using':** David Gelles, 'Gregg Renfrew of Beautycounter on Toxic Chemicals and Getting Fired by Messenger,' *New York Times*, Nov. 21, 2018.

109 **one out of three beauty products:** Elizabeth Paton, 'The Dirt on Clean Beauty,' *New York Times*, Jan. 4, 2023.

Notes

109 'Our job is to create': Kara McGrath, 'Did Clean Beauty Go Too Far?,' *Allure*, Aug. 10, 2023.

DRESSING TO BE WELL

111 'internal organs being displaced': Rebecca N. Mitchell, ed., *Fashioning the Victorians: A Critical Sourcebook* (London: Bloomsbury, 2018), 82.

112 a thirty-two-year-old professional woman: Amy Wallace, 'Chip Wilson, Lululemon Guru, Is Moving On,' *New York Times*, Feb. 2, 2015.

113 'Women's lives changed immediately': Hayley Peterson, '8 Outrageous Remarks by Lululemon Founder Chip Wilson,' *Business Insider*, Dec. 10, 2013.

114 the opportunity to take a free self-help course: Bryan Urstadt, 'Lust for Lulu,' *New York*, July 4, 2009.

114 'It's the first time I've heard': Danielle Sacks, 'Lululemon's Cult of Selling,' *Fast Company*, April 1, 2009.

114 'found no evidence of seaweed': Louise Story, '"Seaweed" Clothing Has None, Tests Show,' *New York Times*, Nov. 14, 2007.

114 one of its chief assets, its 'secret sauce': Kim Bhasin and Ashley Lutz, 'Here's What's So Special About Lululemon's "Luon" Fabric,' *Business Insider*, May 19, 2013.

117 The Global Wellness Institute predicts: Rona Berg, 'The Future of Wellness: New Data on Wellness Travel, Mental Wellness,' *Forbes*, Nov. 10, 2023.

GLOW LIFESTYLE

124 'They told me they needed somebody younger': Linda Wells, 'Isabella Rossellini on Living Well and Aging Gracefully,' *New York*, May 5, 2016.

PART III: SPIRIT AND SOUL

130 In my grandparents' generation: Frank Newport,

'Percentage of Christians in U.S. Drifting Down, but Still High,' *Gallup News*, Dec. 24, 2015, news.gallup.com.

130 **The number of adult Americans:** Pew Forum on Religion & Public Life, 'U.S. Religious Landscape Study' (Washington, D.C.: Pew Research Center, 2008), www.pewforum.org.

131 **70 percent of Americans describe:** Becka Alper et al., 'Spirituality Among Americans,' Pew Research Center, Dec. 7, 2023, www.pewforum.org.

SOUL

132 **'Millennials are flocking to a host':** Angie Thurston and Casper ter Kuile, 'How We Gather,' Sacred Design Lab, Cambridge, Mass., April 2015.

136 **'overcoming the issues in our tissues':** Stacey Griffith, *Two Turns from Zero: Pushing to Higher Fitness Goals – Converting Them to Life Strength* (New York: HarperCollins, 2017), 10.

137 **'Ritual is so much about intention':** Tara Isabella Burton, 'CrossFit Is My Church,' *Vox*, Sept. 10, 2018.

139 **'The stuff that happened':** Michelle Boorstein, 'Peloton Makes Toning Your Glutes Feel Spiritual. But Should Jesus Be Part of the Experience?,' *Washington Post*, Feb. 8, 2021.

139 **'growing health epidemic':** Vivek Murthy, 'Work and the Loneliness Epidemic,' *Harvard Business Review*, Sept. 26, 2017, hbr.org.

139 **'Loneliness is far more than':** Vivek Murthy, *Our Epidemic of Loneliness and Isolation: The U.S. Surgeon General's Advisory on the Healing Effects of Social Connection and Community*, Office of the U.S. Surgeon General, 2023, www.hhs.gov.

Notes

EXERCISE

143 **'Every major figure of the postwar'**: Kate Bowler, *Blessed: A History of the American Prosperity Gospel* (Oxford: Oxford University Press, 2013), 167–68.

144 **'Dear God... Please free me'**: Marianne Williamson, *A Course in Weight Loss: 21 Spiritual Lessons for Surrendering Your Weight Forever* (New York: Hay House, 2010), 14.

144 **'you don't really mean to be grasping'**: Williamson, *Course in Weight Loss*, 150.

145 **'Bitch, you have this job'**: Devon Ivie, 'Why Is Gwyneth Paltrow's Go-To Quote About Bitching Out a Yoga Studio Employee?,' *Vulture*, Jan. 5, 2019.

145 **'I cannot read a single sentence'**: J. J. Clarke, *Oriental Enlightenment: The Encounter Between Asian and Western Thought* (New York: Routledge, 1997), 86.

146 **In the 1960s, more than forty television stations**: Alistair Shearer, *The Story of Yoga: From Ancient India to the Modern West* (London: Hurst, 2020), 214.

146 **'If you are a young soul'**: Vanessa Grigoriadis, 'Flex Appeal,' *New York*, Nov. 19, 2001.

147 **'coming up into a plank position'**: Rina Raphael, 'Where Group Prayer Meets Group Fitness,' *New York Times*, May 19, 2020.

148 **'My soul was tugged'**: Oprah Winfrey, host, *Oprah's Super Soul*, 100 series, 'Oprah and Angela Manuel Davis: Your Life in Focus,' OWN Podcasts, April 22, 2020.

148 **'Forgiveness is a big deal to Jesus'**: Nadia Bolz-Weber, *Pastrix: The Cranky, Beautiful Faith of a Sinner and Saint* (New York: Worthy, 2013), 148.

SELF-LOVE

151 **'The invitation in this pain'**: Glennon Doyle, *Love Warrior: A Memoir* (New York: Flatiron Books, 2016), 164.

151 **'I can feel that the intention'**: Ariel Foxman, 'Glennon Doyle and Abby Wambach Share Their California Home,' *Architectural Digest*, May 24, 2022.

151 **'My job is to write'**: Macaela MacKenzie, 'For Glennon Doyle, Self-Care Is Not Wearing Makeup – or Pants,' *Glamour*, May 27, 2020.

152 **'In a society that says'**: Brené Brown, *The Gifts of Imperfection: Let Go of Who You Think You're Supposed to Be and Embrace Who You Are* (New York: Simon & Schuster, 2010), 41.

152 **'From the time we're born'**: Sarah Larson, 'Brené Brown's Empire of Emotion,' *New Yorker*, Oct. 25, 2021.

153 **Cleo Wade's best-known work**: Cleo Wade, *Heart Talk: Poetic Wisdom for a Better Life* (New York: Simon & Schuster, 2018), 188.

156 **'We realized,' Rice told**: Katherine Rosman, 'SoulCycle Without the Bike: Here Comes Peoplehood,' *New York Times*, May 7, 2022.

CULT

160 **the tale of Sarma Melngailis**: Dana Schuster and Georgett Roberts, 'The Downfall of NYC's Hottest Vegan,' *New York Post*, May 22, 2016.

160 **she was revealed to have suggested**: Dana Schuster, 'Sarma Melngailis Had a Steamy Affair with Her Married Lawyer,' *New York Post*, Jan. 12, 2019.

OUTSIDE OF EXERCISE

162 **the global astrology industry**: Sydney Page, 'Young People Are Flocking to Astrology. But It Comes with Risks,' *Washington Post*, June 13, 2023.

163 **'Ms. Nicholas's words still covered me'**: Jazmine Hughes, 'Your Favorite Internet Astrologer Wrote a Book,' *New York Times*, Jan. 4, 2020.

Notes

164 **'You go to some crystal shops':** Zan Romanoff, 'Breakfast with Hollywood's Favorite Crystal Healer,' *Bon Appétit*, May 9, 2017.

PART IV: PURE

169 **All the COVID in the world:** Christian Yates, 'Why All the World's Coronavirus Would Fit in a Can of Cola,' BBC.com, Feb. 10, 2021.

170 **The man was unaware that black licorice:** Maria Cramer, 'A Man Died After Eating a Bag of Black Licorice Every Day,' *New York Times*, Sept. 26, 2020.

171 **'a doctor must seek out old wives':** Paul Strathern, *Mendeleyev's Dream: The Quest for the Elements* (New York: Pegasus Books, 2019), 74.

171 **'All things are poison':** Brendon Evans, 'Paracelsus: Father of Toxicology, Brother of General Practice,' *Australian Journal of General Practice* 52, no. 6 (June 2023): 333.

172 **4handbook for new immigrants:** Sarah Horton and Judith Barker, "Stains' on Their Self-Discipline: Public Health, Hygiene, and the Disciplining of Undocumented Immigrant Parents in the Nation's Internal Borderlands,' *American Ethnologist* 36, no. 4 (Nov. 2009): 784–98.

CLEANSE

174 **The air we breathe:** From an interview on Goop: https://goop.com/wellness/ detox/clean/?srsltid=AfmBOopHiOz9ZAogES79nPp7Wn7yO4G9ci6Ldk1a lz9Dvp6ps-PbgrX.

175 **In 2006 a developmental biologist:** Jerrold Heindel, 'History of the Obesogen Field: Looking Back to Look Forward,' *Frontiers in Endocrinology* 10 (Jan. 2019): 14, www.frontiersin.org.

177 **cayenne pepper dilates blood vessels:** Peter Glickman,

The Master Cleanse Coach: Expert Coaching for You and Your Friends (Clearwater, Fla.: Peter Glick-man, 2013), 56.

177 he described himself as woozy: Jeffrey Steingarten, 'Mr. Clean: Jeffrey Steingarten Puts the Master Cleanse to the Test,' *Vogue*, May 1, 2012.

178 'The "cleanse and detoxify" idea is nonsense': Amanda Chan, '5 Experts Answer: Is There Such Thing as a Healthy Juice Cleanse,' Live Science, May 30, 2013, www.livescience.com.

179 Juice cleanses got popular: Courtney Rubin, 'Cleansing's Dirty Secret,' *Marie Claire*, April 26, 2013.

184 the subject of one scientific study: A. Golay et al., 'Similar Weight Loss with Low-Energy Food Combining or Balanced Diets,' *International Journal of Obesity and Related Metabolic Disorders* 24, no. 4 (April 2000): 492–96.

185 I couldn't help thinking of another pathology: Steven Bratman, 'Orthorexia vs. Theories of Healthy Eating,' *Eating and Weight Disorders* 22 (2017): 381–85.

185 a popular wellness lifestyle blogger: Bee Wilson, 'Why We Fell for Clean Eating,' *Guardian*, Aug. 11, 2017.

185 'What I was experiencing': Jordan Younger, *Breaking Vegan: One Woman's Journey from Veganism, Extreme Dieting, and Orthorexia to a More Balanced Life* (Beverly, Mass.: Fair Winds Press, 2015), 32.

ENVIRONMENT

188 The FDA has approved: Ben Tracy, 'FDA Hasn't Approved Some Food Additives in Decades,' *CBS Evening News*, Feb. 21, 2023.

188 These are among the forty thousand plus: Lauren Zanolli and Mark Oliver, 'Explained: The Toxic Threat in Everyday Products, from Toys to Plastic,' *Guardian*, May 22, 2019.

Notes

190 Kobi Karp, an architect in Miami: Debra Kamin, 'Meet the New Caregiver: Your Home,' *New York Times*, Sept. 9, 2020.

191 the company could not scientifically: Reeves Wiedeman, 'The Magic Molecule,' *New York*, March 16, 2021.

192 'I think at this point now': Sam Dean, 'The Luxury Air Business Is Booming – as Many Californians Struggle to Breathe,' *Los Angeles Times*, Sept. 23, 2020.

192 'The better your air': Candace Jackson, 'How Fresh Air Became the Must-Have Home Upgrade,' *Town & Country*, Aug. 11, 2020.

193 'Can anyone believe it': Rachel Carson, *Silent Spring* (New York: Houghton Mifflin, 1962), 8.

193 'If the Bill of Rights contains': Carson, *Silent Spring*, 12–13.

194 'When one is concerned with': Carson, *Silent Spring*, 189.

195 Asthma rates among lower-income Americans: Roni Caryn Rabin, 'Poor Americans More Likely to Have Respiratory Problems, Study Finds,' *New York Times*, May 28, 2021.

ALL NATURAL

196 'The more artificial a human environment': Wendell Berry, *Home Economics: Fourteen Essays* (Berkeley, Calif.: Counterpoint Press, 1987), 7.

198 in 1870, two-thirds of Germans: Oliver Grant, *Migration and Inequality in Germany, 1870–1913* (Oxford: Oxford University Press, 2005), 61.

199 'Wander Barefoot': Frank Lipman and Danielle Claro, *The New Health Rules: Simple Changes to Achieve Whole-Body Wellness* (New York: Artisan Books, 2014), 165.

POLITICS

202 'The world of wellness': Mira Miller, 'Naomi Klein on the Link Between Wellness Influencers and Far-Right Propagandists,' *Globe and Mail*, Oct. 5, 2023.

203 'We recognize that separating humanity': Janet Biehl and Peter Staudenmaier, *Ecofascism Revisited: Lessons from the German Experience* (Porsgrunn, Norway: New Compass Press, 2011), 10.

204 'We started to hear': Miller, 'Naomi Klein on the Link Between Wellness Influencers and Far-Right Propagandists.'

204 made headlines when she opened Lucky Lee's: Sharon Otterman, 'A White Restaurateur Advertised "Clean" Chinese Food. Chinese-Americans Had Something to Say About It,' *New York Times*, April 12, 2019.

VACCINES AND THE RABBIT HOLE

207 'That morning my reading': Eula Biss, *On Immunity: An Inoculation* (Minneapolis: Graywolf Press, 2014), 129.

208 'I was not comforted that the oil': Biss, *On Immunity*, 130.

209 the babes to sprout little hooves: Jess McHugh, 'The World's First Anti-vaccination Movement Spread Fears of Half-Cow Babies,' *Washington Post*, Nov. 14, 2021.

210 'I was unwilling to vaccinate': Lisa Miller, 'Measles for the One Percent,' *New York*, May 29, 2019.

210 'We're gonna be the antidote': Tess Owen, 'Unvaccinated TikTokers Are Calling Themselves "Purebloods,"' *Vice News*, Sept. 15, 2021.

211 'normalize eating dirt': 'A Dirt Detox: What's It All About?,' Poosh, https://poosh.com/dirt-detox/.

212 allowing her children to play and crawl: Katie Wells, 'Why Kids Need Dirt,' Nov. 22, 2013, *Wellness Mama*, https://wellnessmama.com/health/kids-need-dirt/.

Notes

212 **'Can you make money'**: Cory Stieg, 'Doctors Are Now Transplanting Poop – & It's Saving Lives,' *Refinery29*, May 2, 2019, www.refinery29.com.

212 **issued a warning when, in 2019**: Andrew Jacobs, 'How Contaminated Stool Stored in a Freezer Left a Fecal Transplant Patient Dead,' *New York Times*, Oct. 30, 2019.

212 **'My fatigue had lifted'**: Carrot Quinn, 'How DIY Fecal Transplant Cured My IBS and Chronic Fatigue (with Updates at the End).' *Carrot Quinn*, May 15, 2020, carrotquinn.com/2017/07/09/how-diy-fecal-transplant-has-so-far-cured-my-ibs-and-chronic-fatigue-with-monthly-updates/.

213 **'I looked around me'**: Carrot Quinn, 'How DIY Fecal Transplant Cured My IBS and Chronic Fatigue,' July 9, 2017, https://carrotquinn.com/2017/07/09/ how-diy-fecal-transplant-has-so-far-cured-my-ibs-and-chronic-fatigue-with-monthly-updates/.

CLEANING AS RITE

215 **'From the moment you start tidying'**: Marie Kondo, *The Life-Changing Magic of Tidying Up: The Japanese Art of Decluttering and Organizing* (Berkeley, Calif.: Ten Speed Press, 2010), 21.

215 **'putting your house in order'**: Kondo, *The Life-Changing Magic of Tidying Up*, 127.

215 **'When you stand under a waterfall'**: Kondo, *The Life-Changing Magic of Tidying Up*, 57.

216 **'As the spring freshets born'**: Joseph Pilates, *Return to Life Through Contrology* (Miami, Fla.: Pilates Method Alliance, 1945), 21.

217 **'fostering creativity, calmness, and cooperation'**: Ann Dooley, *Simplejoywithann*, www.simplejoywithann.com.

217 **'Having a tidy home'**: Lisa Tselebidis, *Lisa Tselebidis*, Oct. 9, 2024, www.lisatselebidis.com/.

MEDITATION/MINDFULNESS

225 **'beautiful serenity and selfless connection'**: Susan Donaldson James, 'Russell Brand Does Stand-Up for Transcendental Meditation,' ABCNews.com, Nov. 29, 2011.

225 **'game changer… neuro pathways open'**: Eviana Hartman, 'What Is Transcendental Meditation? Katy Perry's Teacher Explains Hollywood's Favorite Pathway to Inner Peace,' *Vogue*, April 14, 2017.

225 **'It's a kick start for your day'**: 'Jennifer Aniston Talks Inner Circle and Beauty Missteps,' PopSugar TV, March 25, 2014.

225 **'it's like a [phone] charger'**: 'Jerry Seinfeld, Bob Roth, and George Stephanopoulos Talk Transcendental Meditation,' *Good Morning America*, ABC, Dec. 13, 2012.

225 **'Meditation is as important as lifting weights'**: Alyssa Roenigk, 'Lotus Pose on Two,' ESPNMag.com, Aug. 21, 2013.

228 **'I saw in a flash'**: Robert Booth, 'Master of Mindfulness, Jon Kabat-Zinn: "People Are Losing Their Minds. That Is What We Need to Wake Up To,"' *Guardian*, Oct. 22, 2017.

228 **'I bent over backwards to structure it'**: Booth, 'Master of Mindfulness, Jon Kabat-Zinn.'

229 **'has the potential to ignite'**: 'Jon Kabat-Zinn: The Mindfulness Revolution,' *Insights at the Edge Podcast with Tami Simon*, Oct. 22, 2019.

229 **'We are in this moment'**: Nellie Bowles, 'Jack Dorsey Is Gwyneth Paltrow for Silicon Valley,' *New York Times*, May 2, 2019.

230 **'in mindful competition with each other'**: Hilary Potkewitz, 'Headspace vs. Calm: The Meditation Battle

Notes

That's Anything but Zen,' *Wall Street Journal*, Dec. 15, 2018.

235 **'Maharaji seemed always to be absorbed':** Daniel Goleman and Richard J. Davidson, *Altered Traits: Science Reveals How Meditation Changes Your Mind, Brain, and Body* (New York: Avery, 2018), 21–22.

235 **'The fact that meditation':** Miguel Farias and Catherine Wikholm, *The Buddha Pill: Can Meditation Change You?* (London: Watkins, 2015), 213.

236 **'Rather than applying mindfulness':** Ronald Purser, *McMindfulness: How Mindfulness Became the New Capitalist Spirituality* (London: Watkins, 2019), 22

TRIPPING

239 **'There had been forty thousand research participants':** Michael Pollan, *How to Change Your Mind: What the New Science of Psychedelics Teaches Us About Consciousness, Dying, Addiction, Depression, and Transcendence* (New York: Penguin Press, 2018), 141–42.

WHAT ABOUT MEN?

242 **American women tend to outlive:** Azeen Ghorayshi, 'An "Unsettling" Drop in Life Expectancy for Men,' *New York Times*, Nov. 13, 2023.

243 **'While we all love a sculpted guy':** Mackenzie Pearson, 'Why Girls Love the Dad Bod,' *Odyssey*, March 30, 2015.

243 **'As long as you're not taking':** John Jannuzzi, 'What Is Dad Bod, and Do You Have It?,' *GQ*, April 30, 2015.

243 **'Why are so many smart women':** Jessica Knoll, 'Smash the Wellness Industry,' *New York Times*, June 8, 2019.

245 **'Like, I'm a guy':** Interview with the author.

BIOHACKING

248 a three-hundred-pound computer engineer: Gordy Megroz, 'Buttered Coffee Could Make You Invincible. And This Man Very Rich,' *Bloomberg Businessweek*, April 21, 2015.

248 'maximizing the potential of which the individual': Dunn, *High-Level Wellness*, 4–5.

250 'steals your mental edge': Chris Gayomali, 'Read This Before You Spend $19 on Bulletproof Coffee Beans,' *Fast Company*, Jan. 23, 2015.

252 Faguet has regular assignations: Stefanie Marsh, 'Extreme Biohacking: The Tech Guru Who Spent $250,000 Trying to Live Forever,' *Guardian*, Sept. 21, 2018.

254 'I wanted to go from good to great': Kristen V. Brown, 'This Guy Injected His Dick with Stem Cells to Try to Make It Bigger,' *Gizmodo*, Feb. 28, 2018.

254 'I'm pretty careful with what I stick up my ass': Arielle Pardes, 'Wellness Influencers Sell False Promises as Health Fears Soar,' *Wired*, April 3, 2020.

256 'our lack of sleep': Matthew Walker, *Why We Sleep: Unlocking the Power of Sleep and Dreams* (New York: Scribner, 2017), 323.

256 'not sleeping enough, which for a portion': Walker, *Why We Sleep*, 188–89.

258 'I thought I was killing it': Julie Mazziotta, 'Gwyneth Paltrow and Kim Kardashian Are in a Tense Competition – over Who Gets More Sleep!,' *People*, Aug. 31, 2021.

259 'healthcare providers should not offer': Robert M. Kwee and Thomas C. Kwee, 'Whole-Body MRI for Preventive Health Screening: A Systematic Review of the Literature,' *Journal of Magnetic Resonance Imaging* 50 (Nov. 2019): 1489–503.

NOTES

IMMORTALITY

265 'enjoy up to a 3 times better chance': Dan Buettner, *The Blue Zones: Lessons for Living Longer from People Who've Lived the Longest* (Washington, D.C.: National Geographic Society, 2008), 3.

266 'The proposition that we can live': Tad Friend, 'Silicon Valley's Quest to Live Forever,' *New Yorker*, March 27, 2017.

267 'has produced near perfect health': Editors, 'Bryan Johnson Sold His Company to PayPal for $800 Million. Now, He's Spending $2 Million a Year to Stay Young Forever – No Cheat Days Allowed,' *Fortune*, July 14, 2023.

267 injected himself with his teenage son's blood plasma: Shannon Thaler, ''No Benefits Detected' from Swapping Blood with His Son, Bryan Johnson Says,' *New York Post*, July 11, 2023.

268 'Our language on this matter': S. Jay Olshansky, Leonard Hayflick, and Bruce A. Carnes, 'Position Statement on Human Aging,' *Journals of Gerontology* 57 (Aug. 2002): 292–97.

CONCLUSION

271 'Though our vigilant pursuit': Carol-Ann Farkas, ''Tons of Useful Stuff': Defining Wellness in Popular Magazines,' *Studies in Popular Culture* 33 (Fall 2010): 113–32.

273 'Resolved, not to talk about myself': Joan Jacobs Brumberg, *The Body Project: An Intimate History of American Girls* (New York: Random House, 1997), xxi.

273 'I will try to make myself better': Brumberg, *The Body Project*, xxi.

INDEX

ABC News 160, 230
Abortion 79–80
ACLU 161
activewear (athleisure) 111, 115–7
Adams, Eric 164
Adaptogens 10, 201, 268
Adidas 115
Adler, Bill 63
Advantia Health 53
Aerie 99
Aerobics 137, 141–2, 262
Ahluwalia, Waris 55
AIDS 244
AIRE 214
air purifiers 173, 191
Alcoholics Anonymous 83
Allen, Woody 34
Allied Market Research 162
All-of-a-Kind Family (Taylor) 172
Alloy 67, 69
Allure 109
Alo Yoga 116
Alpha Power 201
Altered Traits (Goleman and Davidson) 235
Alzheimer's 107, 189
Amazon 48, 50, 169, 188, 215, 226, 246
Amazon Prime Video 98

American College of Preventive Medicine 259
American College of Radiology 259
American Kale Association 17
American Medical Association 58
American Psychiatric Association 239
Anderson, Tracy 154
Anderson, Wes 55
Angelou, Maya 70
Aniston, Jennifer 225
Annie Hall (film) 34
anthroposophic ideas 209
Anti-vaxxers 210
Anusara yoga 160
Apiece Apart 121–3
apple cider vinegar (ACV) 57–9, 163
Architectural Digest 46, 151–2
Aristotle 104
Arzon, Robin 134
Asbestos 194, 206
Ashram wellness retreat 117
Ashwagandha 22, 201, 271
Asprey, Dave 248–50, 254, 257, 265
Asthma 191, 195, 278
Astrology 162–3
Athleta 116

INDEX

Atkin, Douglas 114
Atlantic 105
A to Z of D-Toxing (Gushée) 206
Atwood, Margaret 200
Avena sativa 201
Axe Body Spray 95
Ayahuasca 133, 241
Ayurveda 36, 175

Bacon, Amanda Chantal 14, 201–2
Bacon, Kevin 41
Bad Vegan (TV show) 160
Bakker, Jim 143
Bakker, Tammy Faye 143
Balenciaga 115
Ball, Allie 53
Baltimore Longitudinal Study of Aging 30
Barrymore, Drew 67
Baudhuin, John 134
Baywatch (film) 27
Beautycounter 108–9
Beckham, David 260
Believercise 143
Beloved 214
Berry, Halle 225
Berry, Wendell 196
Berzin, Robin 44–7, 52, 186
Betty Boop, M.D. (short film) 61
Beyoncé 17, 115, 177
Beyond the Scale initiative 96
Bezos, Jeff 251, 266
Bhagavad Gita 145
Biden, Joe 129, 139
Bieber, Hailey 200
Bigorexia 244
Big Pharma 272
Billions (TV show) 215
Bilz, Friedrich 199
Biohacking 221, 248–60, 269
Biomonitoring 188

biophilic design 47–8, 115
Biss, Eula 207–8
Black Americans 30–1, 84, 195, 209
Black Panther Party (BPP) 80–1
Bland, Jeffrey 40–1
Blessed (Bowler) 143
Bloom, Orlando 59
Bloomer, Amelia 112, 116
BluePrint 176–80
Blue Zones 264–9, 280–1
Blue Zones (Buettner) 264
body positivity 90, 96, 99, 101, 111, 175
Body Project, The (Bruberg) 273
body scan 259–60
Bo'ed, Tae 141
Bolz-Weber, Nadia 148
Bono 55, 108
Botox 50, 224
Bouley, David 42
Bowler, Kate 143–4
Boyle, T. C. 35
BPAs 54, 175, 180
Bragg, Patricia 58–9
Bragg, Paul 58–9
Bragg Health Crusade 58
brain fog 47, 68, 190, 213, 241
Brain Force Plus 201
Brand, Russell 225
Bratman, Steven 185
breast milk 21, 136
breathing technique 133, 146, 278
Brekhman, Israel 201
Bridal Glow vitamins 91
Brin, Sergey 266
British Medical Journal 66
Bronx Veterans Affairs Medical Center 99
Brown, Bobbi 91, 275
Brown, Brené 131, 151–3
Brumberg, Joan Jacobs 273

304

Buddha Pill, The (Farias and Wikholm) 235
Buddhism 155
Buettner, Dan 264–8
Bulletproof coffee 250
Bündchen, Gisele 97, 225
Burke, Tarana 152
Burning Man 52
Burroughs, Stanley 177
Burt's Bees 192
Bush, George H. W. 34
ButYouDontLookSick.com blog 73

Calico (California Life Company) 266
Calm app 230
Campbell, Naomi 98, 118
Cancer Alley 195
CAP Beauty 92
Carlyle Group 109
Carnegie, Dale 83
Carnegie Foundation 29
Carson, Rachel 193–5
Catholics 129, 142
Caulfield, Timothy 59–60
CBD 2, 49, 173, 240–1, 263, 268
celiac disease 15, 196–7
Center for Human Sleep Science 256
Centers for Disease Control (CDC) 74, 84
Chanel 41, 99, 123
Chansley, Jacob (QAnon Shaman) 202
Chapman, Jake 15
Chapman, John (Johnny Appleseed) 57–8
Chapo, El 160
Cheiro 162
Chenot, Henri 119
Chenot Palace 119

Chiang Kai-shek, Madame 146
Chicago World's Fair 145
Childbirth 49, 84
China, ancient 162
Chinese medicine 36, 91, 197
Chloé 99
Chopra, Deepak 54, 190
Christianity 57–8, 130, 137, 142–50
chronic illness 72–7
ChurchFIT 147
Churchill, Winston 162
Clairol 92
Claro, Danielle 199
Class, the 153, 158
Clean Market 173
clean products 188–9
Clean program 180
cleansing and cleanliness 64, 174–87
Clemson University 243
Cleveland, Grover 162
Cleveland Clinic 43, 74, 249
Center for Functional Medicine 43
Clevr Blends 54
Clinton, Chelsea 54
Clostridioides difficile 212
Cocaine 61, 133, 160, 183, 249
Collagen 19, 91, 276
Colonics 10, 118, 181–6
Columbia University 44, 66
Medical School 29–31, 44, 101, 228
Committee for Skeptical Inquiry 62
Confucius 162
continuous glucose monitors (CGMs) 22, 258–9
Controlled Substances Act () 240
Contrology 216
Cordyceps 14, 201

INDEX

Corexit 208
Corpus deodorant 107
CoStar 163
Costco 16
Couric, Katie 225
'Course, The,' 153
Course in Miracles, A (Williamson) 144
Course in Weight Loss (Williamson) 144
COVID- 18, 21, 55–6, 65, 84, 130, 139, 163, 169, 188–191, 201–2, 210, 242, 254
COVID vaccine 56, 202, 210
Crave 106
Crosley, Sloane 27
CrossFit 137, 148, 159
CrossFit Faith 148
Crystal Academy of Advanced Healing Arts 164
Crystals 62, 131, 158, 162–5
Culting of Brands, The (Atkin) 114
Cutler, Elizabeth 155

Dada Daily snacks 124
Daily Beast 74
Dalai Lama 238
Dame 106
Dancy, Hugh 105
Danguin, Pascal 95
David, Ned 266
Davidson, Richard J. 234–5
Davis, Angela Manuel 148
Daytime Emmy Awards 65
DDT 174, 193–5
Deepwater Horizon oil spill 208
DeGeneres, Ellen 225
Democratic Party 144
Deodorants 107, 172, 189, 277–8
D'Ercole, Christine 140
Detoxification 54, 117–9, 173–8, 181, 189, 200, 211–6

Devi, Indra (Eugenie Peterson) 145–6
Devil Wears Prada, The (film) 19
Diamant, Anita 214
diatomaceous earth 211
Diaz, Cameron 69
digital detoxes 181
Dior, Christian 115
Doctors Who Rock gala 210
Dôen 121–2
Doing Harm (Dusenbery) 76
Dominus, Susan 68
Dooley, Ann 217
Dooley Method 217
dopamine detox 181
Doppelganger (Klein) 202
Dorsey, Jack 229, 251–2
Dove Campaign for Real Beauty 95
Downer, Carol 79–80
Doyle, Glennon 150–1
Dr. Barbara Sturm's Glow Drops 90
Dreamgirls (musical) 177
Dr. Google 249
Dr. Oz Show, The (TV show) 65–6, 206
Dr. Scholl's 58
dry brushing 90
Dudum, Andrew 245–6
Dunham, Lena 72, 225
Dunkin' Donuts 16
Dunn, Halbert L. 36–7, 240, 248
Durant, Kevin 229
Dusenbery, Maya 75–7, 253

Eastwood, Clint 225
Eat, Pray, Love (Gilbert) 150
Ebers Papyrus 104, 182
Edna ad campaign 92, 110
Egypt, ancient 162, 182
Ehlers-Danlos syndrome 72–3

Eight Weeks to Optimum Health (Weil) 38
Einkorn 197
Einstein, Albert 217–8
Elders, Joycelyn 247
election of 2016 157
Elemis's Superfood Glow Priming Moisturiser 90
Eleven Eleven clinic 41
e.l.f.'s Halo Glow 90
Elle 14, 210, 225, 230
Ellis, Susie 262–3
Elsesser, Paloma 99
Emerson, Ralph Waldo 145
Eng, John 100
Environmental Protection Agency 188, 195
environmental wellness 189, 194
enVy 256
Epstein, Jeffrey 98
Erewhon 200
Essential Guide to Becoming Superhuman, The (Greenfield) 253
Estée Lauder 91
European Congress of Psychology 164
Evernow 69
Evolution products 91, 252
Exendin- 100

Fabletics 116
Face, The 15
Facebook 74
Faguet, Serge 252
Fair & Lovely skin lightening Creams 95
Faithercise 143
Fallon, Jimmy 59, 110
Fanon, Frantz 81
Farias, Miguel 235
Farkas, Carol-Ann 271
fashion. *See also* activewear 12–4, 51, 55, 97–9, 115–6, 120–5, 158, 263
Fast Company 114
fasting, intermittent 14, 58, 143–4, 175, 179, 251
Fasting (Franklin) 144
Fauci, Dr. 210
fecal transplants 173, 212
Fegan, MacKenzie Chung 204
Felix Gray 257
feminist movement 79–80, 111
Feminist Women's Health Center 80
Fendi 99
Fenty collection 116
Ferguson, Rosemary 15
Ferguson, Sarah 96
Finding Ultra (Roll) 254
Fitbit 250
fitness industry 111–13, 130–65, 180
Fitzgerald, Janet 133, 136, 158–9
Flat Tummy shakes 125
Flexner, Abraham 29–31, 34, 36, 40, 60, 73
Flint, Michigan 195
Flow 253
Floyd, George 130
Foley, John 139
Fonda, Jane 34
Food and Drug Administration (FDA) 108, 174–5, 188–9, 192, 208, 212
food combining diet 184–5
food sensitivities 28, 255
Forbes 55
Ford, Tom 115
Fordham University 149
Forward Station dance studio 157, 280
Franklin, Jentezen 144
Franklin, Benjamin 83

INDEX

Free Health Clinic 81
Friend, John 160
Friend, Tad 266
Fulenwider, Anne 67–9
functional medicine 18, 40–5, 53–6, 73, 92, 175, 255

Galeota, Isabella Capece 15
Gap 41, 115
Garbo, Greta 146
Gardenburger 58
Garner, Jennifer 99
General Mills 229
Gerbic, Susan 62
Germany 118, 198–9
Geronimus, Arline 81–3
Gershon, Michael 178
Gilbert, Elizabeth 150
Ginseng 201
Glamglow's Glowstarter 90
Glamour 151
Glickman, Peter 177
Global Wellness Institute 11, 117, 262
Global Wellness Summit (GWS) 262, 267
Globe and Mail 202, 204
Glossier's Super Glow 90
Glow 90–6, 102–7, 117, 124, 175, 251
Gluten 15–6, 54, 124, 143, 185, 196–7, 263, 274
GNC 58
Goddess Glow Collagen Peptides 91
Godfrey, Jay 239
Goldberg, Jonathan 'Johnny G' 134
Goldberg, Susan 215
Golden Door spa 262
Golden State Warriors 226
Goldman Sachs 229, 238

Goleman, Daniel 234–5
Golovanoff, Alexandra 15–6
Good Life magazine 65
Good Morning America (TV show) 230
Google 53, 63, 65, 121, 235, 249, 266
Goop 16, 59–62, 67, 91, 103–5, 109, 120, 173–4, 212–4, 226, 230, 246
  Double-Sided Wand Vibrator 105
  Everyday Glow multivitamin 91
  Four Keys to Mindful Parenting 226
  Made You Blush kit 105
Gordon, Aubrey 57–9, 101
Gore, Al 108
GQ 243
Graham, Ashley 99
Gravity 182
Great Yogurt Conspiracy 80
Greenfield, Ben 253–4
Griffith, Melanie 118
Griffith, Stacey 136
Grigoriadis, Vanessa 146
Guerlain's Abeille Royale Bee Glow 90
Guerrilla Skeptics 62
Guevara, Che 81
Guinness World Records 252
Gunter, Jennifer 60
Gushée, Sopia Ruan 206
Guy, Molly Rosen 122
Gyllenhaal, Maggie 41–2, 105
gym culture 113–8, 135–8, 227, 242–4, 260

Hackd Fitness 260
Hadid, Gigi 97–8
Haggard, Ted 159

Hahnemann, Christian Samuel 198
Hain Celestial Group 179
hair coloring 92
Hamlin's Wizard Oil 61
Handmaid's Tale, The (Atwood) 200
Harris, Dan 227, 230, 234
Harris, Kamala 210
Harvard Business Review 139
Harvard University 37, 40, 234–5
Harvest Bible Chapel, Sport Ministry 144
Haspel, Arielle 204
Hay diet 184
HBO Max 234
Headspace app 230
Healthcare Design 53
Healthy Kitchen, The (Weil) 38
Healthy Living (magazine) 16
Healthy Living (TV show) 144
Heart Talk (Wade) 152
Heller, Sabine 55
Hers 246
Hess, Rudolph 203
High-Level Wellness (Dunn) 37
Hill, Napoleon 83
Hills, The (TV show) 164
Himmler, Heinrich 203
Hims 245–6
Hinduism 36, 145
Hippocrates 36, 104
Hittleman, Richard 146
Hobbes, Michael 57
Hof, Wim 'Iceman,' 252, 255
holistic medicine 32–6, 40–1, 73, 255
HomeCleanse 190
Homeopathy 198
Hooters 48
Hopkins, Anthony 35

hormone replacement therapy (HRT) 68–70
House for All Sinners and Saints 148
Howard University College of Medicine 30
How to Change Your Mind (Pollan) 239
How to Win Friends and Influence People (Carnegie) 83
'How We Gather' (Thurston and ter Kuile) 132, 137
Hubbard method 215
Huffington, Arianna 54, 229
Huffington Post, The 54
Hughes, Jazmine 163
HUM's Hyaluronic Glow Gummies 91
Hunt, Martha 27
Hunter College 125
Hurley, Elizabeth 118
Huss, Erica 179
Huynh, Mélanie 15
Hyman, Dr. Mark 43–5, 119
Hysteria 104
Hysteria (film) 105

Ikaria 265
ImmerseNYC 214
Immortality 262–70
Inconvenient Truth, An (film) 108
India 145, 150, 162, 180, 201, 231
indoor air quality 190–2
induction ovens 191
Industrial Revolution 57, 198
Infowars 200–1
In Goop Health conference () 214
Instagram 14–5, 18, 47, 72, 74, 84, 118, 124, 137, 149–52, 187, 204, 228, 258–9
insulin regulation 100
intention-based mantra 227

INDEX

International Journal of Obesity and Related Metabolic Disorders 184
In the Next Room, or, The Vibrator Play (Ruhl) 105
Invisible Kingdom (O'Rourke) 75
Is Gwyneth Paltrow Wrong about Everything? (Caulfield) 59
I Thought It Was Just Me (Brown) 152
Ivy Park line 115

Jackson, Alicia 69
Jacobs, Gil 182–6
January, attack on Capitol 202
Jay-Z 97
Jazzercise 143
Jimmy Fallon (TV show) 59, 110
Jivamukti 146
Joali Being 119
Jobs, Steve 225
Joe & the Juice 180
John of God 64
Johns Hopkins 29, 68
Johnson, Bryan 266–7
Johnson & Johnson 110, 194
Jones, Alex 200–1
Jones, Mike 160
Judaism 129–30, 142, 172, 214, 239
Judd, Naomi 225
Juice Beauty 109
juice cleanse 176–9
Juice Generation 180
Juice Press 180
Junger, Alejandro 174, 180

Kabat-Zinn, Jon 228–9
Kabbalah 239
Kaiser Family Foundation 84
Kale 17
Kapleau, Philip 228
Kardashian, Khloé 125
Kardashian, Kim 99, 125, 258
Kardashian, Kourtney 211
Karman, Harvey 79
karma yoga 133
Karp, Kobi 190
Kayne, Jennie 121, 123
Kennedy, Jackie 89
Kennedy, Robert F., Jr. 209
Kenneth, Mr. 89–92
Ketamine 221, 237, 239, 241
Khaite 115
Khakpour, Porochista 74, 77
Kickapoo Indian Oil 61
Kilimanjaro 252
King, Billie Jean 151
King, Gayle 70
King, Martin Luther, Jr. 138
Klein, Naomi 202–3
Kloss, Karlie 118
Klum, Heidi 97
Kneipp, Sebastian 199
Kneipp Cure 199
Knoll, Jessica 243
Kondo, Marie 215–7, 275
KonMari method 217
KORA Organics' Turmeric Glow Moisturizer 90
Koroshetz, Kiki 105
Kors, Michael 99
Kotler, Steven 253
Koyfman, Hilary 46
Krishnamacharya, Sri 145
Kriya Yoga 145
Kroll, Nick 27
Kruger, Ben 55
Kruger, Bernard 55
Kuhne, Louis 198
Kundalini meditation 14, 158, 227
Kusama, Yayoi 28

Labracadabra effect 255
Lacy, Andrew 259
Lady's Handbook for Her Mysterious Illness, The (Ramey) 32, 75
Lagerfeld, Karl 116
Lam, Amanda 109
Lamb, Dr. Angela 91
Lancet 209
Lancôme 124–5
Landmark Forum 114
Lanserhof medical spas 118
Larkin, Philip 276
Lauren, Ralph 38, 55, 111
Lavender, Jillian 231
Leary, Timothy 37, 235, 240
Lebensreformers 199, 265
Lee, Azalea 164
Lehmann, Ernst 203
lemonade diet 177
Leoni, Téa 42
Levels CGM 258
Levy, Joyce 159
Libran, Julie de 15
Licorice 170, 172, 213
Life-Changing Magic of Tidying Up, The (Kondo) 215
life coaching 155
life expectancy 106, 242
lifestyle apps 163
Lily, The 112
Lima, Adriana 98
Lincoln Medical Center (Bronx) 42
Lipman, Frank 41–5, 92, 199
Listerine 92
Little Book of Mindfulness, The (Collard) 226
Liv 53
Live Water 195
Lola 192–3
Lorde, Audre 82–4

Louis Vuitton Foundation 15
Louis XI 182
Louis XIV 182
Love, Ally 140, 149
Lovewell, Emma 154
Love Wellness's Good to Glow 91
Love Yoga 121
loving-kindness meditation 227
LSD 147, 237–40
Lucky Lee's 204
Lululemon 112–6
Lumen 258–9
Luria, Sara 214–5
Lutheranism 148
LVMH 116
Ly, Alda 53
Lyme disease 15, 72–5
Lyons, Jenna 118

Maca 14, 201
Macpherson, Elle 210
Madd Dog Athletics 135
Madonna 135, 225
Magic Mountain, The (Mann) 118
Mahendran, Lavanya 121
Mahon, Janine 91
Maines, Rachel 104–5
Maintenance Phase podcast 101
Malin, Greg 192
Mall of America 48
Malone, Sharon 69
Mantra 21, 223, 227, 232–3
Manusmriti 145
Mao Zedong 81
Maples, Marla 262
Mar-a-Lago 262
Marathons 182, 252–6
Marie Antoinette 89, 116
Marie Claire 67, 179
Marijuana 38, 49–50, 237–40
Markle, Meghan 54
Mary Kay cosmetics 108

Index

Maisie Café 16
Massachusetts General Hospital 212
Master Cleanse 177–8
May, Theresa 118
Mayr method 118
Mayyim Hayyim Living Waters 214
McCarthy, Jenny 64–5, 209
McCartney, Paul 225
McCartney, Stella 115
McKinney, Charlotte 27
McKinsey & Company 11
McMindfulness (Purser) 236
medicine, traditional 32–3, 272
medical road shows 63
medical trials 30
Meditation 9–10, 14–5, 38, 92, 121–3, 142, 145, 153–5, 158, 165, 171, 221–40, 269–70, 274–6
meditation apps 230
Meditation for Fidgety Skeptics (Harris) 234
Megachurches 143–4, 159
Meharry Medical College 30
Melngailis, Sarma 160
Melville, Brandy 101
Men 30, 79, 113, 116, 201, 209, 221, 231, 242–54
Menopause 30, 67–71, 106, 222
menstrual extractions 79–80
#MeToo 98, 225
Metrosexuals 244
Microplastics 188, 191
Mikvah 214–5
Milano, Alyssa 27
Miller, Alyssa, 121
Miller, Elizabeth Smith 111
Miller, Michael 223–4, 231–4, 270

Miller, Sienna 41
Miller, Susan 164
Minaj, Nicki 97
Mindfulness 22, 131, 200, 223–236, 251
Mindfulness-Based Stress Reduction (MBSR) 228
Mindfulness for Beginners (Kabat-Zinn) 226
Miracle of Mindfulness (Naht Hanh) 226
Miserandino, Christine 73–4
Missoni 115
Miu Miu 15
Modern Age 50, 269
Molekule 191
Monroe, Marilyn 89, 99
Montag, Heidi 164
Moon Juice 201–2
Moore, Julianne 169
Morris, Kelly 146
Moss, Kate 15, 118
Motherhood 21, 206
Mount Zion Baptist Church (Nashville) 148
MRI 259–60
Mrozinski, Sharon 122
Mullen, Seamus 246
Multiple Risk Factor Intervention Trial (MRFIT) 30
Murthy, Vivek 139
Muse 226
Muslims 142
Mycotoxins 250
Myss, Caroline 60–2
mytheresa.com 117

Naiman, Kristen 123
NARS 103
National Advertising Division 191
National Association of Evangelicals 159

National Institute of Mental Health 38
National Institutes of Health (NIH) 241
National Museum of African American History and Culture 100
National Organization for Women (NOW) 79
Natural Doctor, The 199
natural products 50, 107–8, 172–3, 196–99, 209–16, 263
Nature Boys 199
Naturopath 66, 199
Naylor, R. H. 162
Nazi Party 199, 203
Neem Karoli, Maharaji 235
Net-a-Porter 117
Netflix 158, 160, 260
New Health Rules, The (Lipman and Claro) 199
New Life megachurch 159
New Yorker 95, 266
New York magazine 146, 279
New York Obstetrical Society 31
New York Post 101, 160
New York Times Magazine 62, 68
Nicholas, Chani 163–4
Nicorette 249
Nicoya Peninsula 265
Nidetch, Jean 96
Nike 115
Nixon, Richard 240
Nordstrom 106
North American Menopause Society (NAMS) 68
Novo Nordisk 100
Nushama Psychedelic Wellness Center 238

O, The Oprah Magazine 64
Oak app 257
Obama, Michelle 50, 67, 69, 129, 148, 151
Obesogens 175
Ob-gyns 49, 53, 68–9, 79–80, 207
Ogilvy & Mather 95
oil pulling 180–1
Okinawa 265
Okung, Russell 225
Old Navy 19, 115
Olshan, Claire 124
Onda 108
On Immunity (Bliss) 207
Onion, The 146
opdoen.com 121
OpenBiome 212
Oprah Daily 70
Oprahmag.com 163
Oprah Winfrey Show, The 63–4
Oral Roberts University 148
Organic Avenue 179
Orgasm 9, 103–5, 147, 254
Orgasm (NARS blush) 103–4
O'Rourke, Meghan 31, 44, 46, 75, 77
Orthodox Jews 214
orthorexia nervosa 185
Osho Kundalini meditation 158
Osteen, Joel 143–4
Ostomy Awareness Day 72
Oula Health 54
Oura ring 252, 257
Our Epidemic of Loneliness and Isolation 139
Outdoor Voices 115
OWN network 69
Oz, Dr. 65–7, 206
Ozempic 99–102

INDEX

Pacific Natural (Kayne) 123
Paltrow, Gwyneth 16, 41–2, 59–61, 69, 109–110, 145, 154, 190, 246, 258
Pamer, Kerilynn 92
Parabens 175, 208
Paracelsus 171, 213, 277
Parekh, Rebecca 54
Parliament of Religions 145
Parsley Health 46–7
Parton, Dolly 151
Passler, Dr. 14
Pat's Diet Shake 144
Pattern app 163
Pawson, John 15
Pearson, Mackenzie 243
Peloton 129, 134, 138–140, 149, 154, 158
Peoplehood 155–6
Perry, Katy 59, 197, 225
Perry, Matthew 241
Pesticides 174, 188, 191–5
Peter, Second Epistle of 148
Petit Trianon 89
Philip Morris 19
Phthalates 90, 174–5, 208, 277
Physical (TV show) N/A
Pilates 21, 137, 216, 275, 280
Pilates, Joseph 12, 216
Pinto, Freida 27
Pizza Hut 17
Planned Parenthood 161
Plato 104
Pollan, Michael 238–9
Poor Richard's Almanack (Franklin) 83
Poosh website 211
PopSugar 225
Poverty 81, 134, 143, 189, 195
Praisercise 143–4
Pratt, Spencer 164
Prenuvo 259–60

Princeton University 81
ProLon 180
prosperity gospel 143
Protestantism 143
Psilocybins 237, 240
Psychedelics 10, 37, 237–9, 276
Ptolemy 162
Public Health Service 209
Pueblo, Yung (Diego Perez) 152–3
Purdue Pharma 51–2
Pure Food and Wine 160
Purif 215
purity. *See also* cleansing and Cleanliness 102, 110, 172, 200–3, 213
Purser, Ronald 236

QAnon 202
Quantified Bob 248, 255
QuickTrim 125
Quinn, Carrot 212
Quinoa 184, 194

Racism 81, 195, 203
Radowitz, Steven 239
Rajneesh, Bhagwan Shree 158–9
Ram Dass (formerly Richard Alpert) 235, 238
Ramey, Sarah 32, 75–7
Randhawa, Kirat 155
Raphaell, Katrina 164
Rather, Dan 33–4, 37
Raydiant 48
Reagan, Ronald 34
Real lingerie campaign 99
Redgrave, Lynn 96
Reed, Lou 142
Refinery 212
Reiki 67, 155
relational fitness 155

religion and spirituality 10, 16, 22, 130–1, 137–150, 214, 253
REM sleep 257
Renfrew, Gregg 108
Return to Life through Contrology (Pilates) 216
Rhodiola 201
Rice, Julie 155–6
Rihanna 116
Rise of Superman, The (Kotler) 253
Ritual 21, 123, 131, 137, 143, 153, 161, 165, 214–5, 241
Road to Wellville, The (Boyle) 105
Robertson, Pat 144
Roll, Rich 254
Rolling Stones 118
Roman 129
Ross, Stephen 239
Rossellini, Isabella 124–5
Rothman, Lorraine 80
Rubino, Michael 190
Ruhl, Sarah 105

Sacai 115
Safe (film) 169
Sage + Sound 155

Sakara Life 180
Sakoutis, Zoe 179
Salon 76
Sanctuary app 163
San Francisco State College 236
San Vicente Bungalows 55
Sardinia 265
Sawyer, Diane 230
scalp purification 213–4
Schwimmer, David 129
Scientology 215
Seinfeld, Jerry 225
Self-care 10, 18, 22, 33, 78–85, 89, 92, 107, 117, 121, 131, 150–1, 201–2, 215, 246, 253

Self-help 80–3, 114, 144, 236
Self-Help (Smiles) 82
Self-improvement 117, 143, 151, 242, 273
Self-love 16, 90, 150–7
Self-Realization Fellowship 145
Selye, Hans 201
Semaglutides 100
Sephora 110
Seventeen magazine 165
Seventh Day Adventists 265, 268
sex toys 16, 106
Shaw, Noa 138
Shelton, Herbert M. 184
Shen 103
Shriver, Maria 69–70
Sick (Khakpour) 74–6
Sicksadgirlz (Instagram account) 72
Sildenafil 246
Silence of the Lambs, The (film) 35
Silent Spring (Carson) 193
Simmons, Russell 146–7
Sims, Jess 134
Sinalco 199
Sinclair, Oberon 17
Six Senses resort 43, 119
60 Minutes (tv show) 33
skin care. *See also* glow 107–110
Skin Laundry 173
Sleep 10, 12, 21, 28, 43–4, 51, 54, 83, 103, 118, 123, 160, 170, 192, 207, 216, 221–6, 233–7, 250–9, 264–9, 274–7
SleepLily 192
sleep monitors 257
SlimFast diet bars 95
Sloth's Guide to Mindfulness, A (Mak) 226
smallpox vaccine 199, 208
'Smash the Wellness Industry' (Knoll) 243

INDEX

Smiles, Samuel 82
Snowe, Olympia 30
Sollis Health 27, 55
Somatropin 252
Sontag, Susan 75
SoulCore 147
SoulCycle 129, 132–9, 148, 155–61
Soul Day 134
Spafinder.com 262
spa industry 262
Spinning 134–40, 148
Spirit Rock 229
spiritual but not religious (SBNR) 131
Spiritual Gangster brand 137
Stanton, Elizabeth Cady 112
Steinem, Gloria 151
Steiner, Rudolf 198, 209
Steingarten, Jeffrey 177
Steinman, Joshua 258
Stewart, Martha 38, 123–4
Stiller, Ben 55
Sting 55
Stone, Gunner 164
Story, Louise 114
Stress 81–3, 103, 112–4, 141, 186, 200–1, 224–8, 231, 234–7, 269, 278
Sturm, Barbara 90, 192
Substack 60
Suffering the Silence 76
Suffragists 111–2
Sufis 142
Sunday Service 133
Sundays with Love 149
Sunscreen 109, 278
Super Male Vitality 201
Supplement 9, 13, 18–20, 28, 30, 38, 40–7, 51, 59, 69, 91, 180, 201, 211, 250, 268, 272, 276–8
survival programs 80

Swanson, Gloria 146
Swift, Taylor 97
Swinton, Tilda 164
Swolverine ACV Gummies 59
sympathetic nervous system 278

tampons, organic cotton 192–3
Target 106
Technogym 263
Technology of Orgasm, The (Maines) 104
TED talks 153, 268
Ten Commandments of Health and Wellness (White) 144
Tend dental chain 49
10% Happier (Harris) 230
10 Reasons You Feel Old and Get Fat and Spent (Lipman) 42
ter Kuile, Casper 132, 137, 165
Terrapin Bright Green 48
THC 38, 241
Theragun 105
Think and Grow Rich (Hill) 83
ThirdLove 99
Thistle 180
Thomson, Larissa 108
Thoreau, Henry David 145
Thurston, Angie 132, 137, 165
Tia 53
Tibetan Buddhism 142, 155
Tiffany's 115
TikTok 74, 210, 244
Time 38
Tisch family 155
Title IX 31
Today show 206
Toomey, Taryn 153–4, 158
Toto toilets 190
Toussaint, Alex 140
Toxins 90, 108, 143, 170–1, 177–80, 206–7, 250, 254

Transcendental Meditation 9, 10, 18, 223–5, 274
Transparent (TV show) 215
Travis, John 33, 37
Trellis 50
Trinity (Christian Broadcasting Network) 144
Troon Pacific 192
TrueDark sunglasses 250
Trump, Donald 18, 66, 83, 130, 161, 201, 209–10, 262
Trump, Ivanka 84
Tselebidis, Lisa 217
Turrell, James 15, 227
Tuskegee Study 209
23andMe 266

Unilever 95
U.S. Army 235
U.S. Congress 66
U.S. Senate 66–7
Unity 266
University of Arizona 39
University of California, Irvine 175
University of Massachusetts Medical School 228
University of Michigan 81
University of Pennsylvania 44, 65
University of Puget Sound 40
University of Texas, Austin 152
Urban Institute 84
USDA 259
Us Weekly 99

Vaccines 55–6, 65, 199, 202, 206–13
Vagina Bible, The (Gunter) 60
vaginal washes 106
Vajenda, The (substack) 60
Vanity Fair 146
Vedas 36

Vedic meditation 21, 231–2
Veet waxing strips 93
Vegetarian Lookout 199
Versace 99
Vesper vibrator 106
Veterans Affairs Department 99
Viagra 246
Vibrators 103–6, 120
Victoria's Secret 27, 97–9
Victoria's Secret: The Tour '23 (video) 98
Vipassana meditation 227, 229
Virginia Commonwealth University 84
Viva Mayr clinic 118
Vivamayr spa 14
Vivekananda, Swami 145
Vogue 15, 46, 102, 177, 225
Vora, Ellen 230
Vox 137
VS&Co. 98

Wade, Cleo 152–3
Wakefield, Andrew 209
Waldorf schools 209–10
Walker, Matthew 256
Walker, Stephanie 147–8
Walker, Warren 148
Walmart 16
Wambach, Abby 69, 151
Wang, Alexander 115
War Paint 245
Washington Post 243
water, bottled 195
Watts, Naomi 67, 69, 108
Weathering 81
WebMD 74, 249
We Can Do Hard Things podcast 151
We Care 117
Wegovy 99–100
weight loss 66, 96–103, 117, 125,

Index

134, 144, 175–6, 179, 184, 242, 250, 273
Weight Watchers (WW) 96–7, 100
Weil, Dr. Andrew 37–40
'Welcome to the Menopause Gold Rush' (Larocca) 69
Well, the 42, 54, 92
wellandgood.com 91, 173
Well + Good 59, 103, 206
wellness industry. *See also specific branches* revenues rise of 21, 28, 103, 172, 243, 248, 274
Wellness Mama blog 211
Wellness Moonshot 263
Wellness Resource Center 33
wellness tourism 117
Wells, Katie 211
West, Kanye 97
Westin Hotels 118
Wexler, Tanya 105
Wexner, Les 98
What Doesn't Kill Us (Hof) 252
White, Paula 144
Who Moved My Cheese? (Johnson) 82
Why We Sleep (Walker) 256
Wielding the Lasso of Truth blog 60
Wigan Warriors 245
Wikholm, Catherine 235
Wildfires 188, 191
Wildist's Tangellow 107
Wild One Glow supplements 91
Wild Wild Country (TV show) 158
Williams, Michelle 41–2
Williamson, Marianne 144
Wilshire Boulevard Temple 215
Wilson, Chip 112–4
Wilson, Rebel 118

Winfrey, Oprah 63–71, 96, 100, 151, 177, 225
Witte, Carolyn 53, 55
Wolf, Naomi 202
Womaness Fountain of Glow 91
'Women Have Been Misled About Menopause' (Dominus) 68
Women's Equity Action League 31
Women's Health Initiative 68
Women Who Work (Trump) 84
Wright, Frank Lloyd 48
Wu, Su 122

X (*formerly* Twitter) 229, 258

yeast infections 80
Yoga 13, 15–16, 19, 45, 111–22, 133, 137, 145–7, 159, 185, 227
Yoga for Health (TV show) 146
Yoga Journal 185
Yogananda, Paramahansa 145
yoga pants 111–2, 120
YogaWorks 160
Yost, Felicity 53
You Are Your Best Thing (Brown and Burke) 151
Young and Slim for Life (Lipman) 42
Younger, Jordan 185

You Were Born for This (Nicholas) 163
Yun, Joon 266

Zen Buddhism 142, 228
Zuckerberg, Mark 251

ABOUT THE AUTHOR

Amy Larocca is an award-winning American journalist. Her writing has appeared in the New York Times, Vogue, Town & Country and the London Review of Books, among others. She lives with her family in New York and North London.

amylarocca.com
@amylaroccaauthor

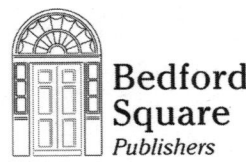

Bedford Square Publishers is an independent publisher of fiction and non-fiction, founded in 2022 in the historic streets of Bedford Square London and the sea mist shrouded green of Bedford Square Brighton.

Our goal is to discover irresistible stories and voices that illuminate our world.

We are passionate about connecting our authors to readers across the globe and our independence allows us to do this in original and nimble ways.

The team at Bedford Square Publishers has years of experience and we aim to use that knowledge and creative insight, alongside evolving technology, to reach the right readers for our books. From the ones who read a lot, to the ones who don't consider themselves readers, we aim to find those who will love our books and talk about them as much as we do.

We are hunting for vital new voices from all backgrounds – with books that take the reader to new places and transform perceptions of the world we live in.

Follow us on social media for the latest Bedford Square Publishers news.

@bedsqpublishers
facebook.com/bedfordsq.publishers
@bedfordsq.publishers

bedfordsquarepublishers.co.uk